Cancer of the Gastrointestinal Tract

Cancer of the Gastrointestinal Tract

A Handbook for Nurse Practitioners

EDITED BY

Davina Porock PhD, RN
Associate Professor, Sinclair School of Nursing,
University of Missouri-Columbia, Missouri

and

Diane Palmer BSc(Hons), RN, PGCE
Lecturer in Nursing, University of Hull, Hull

SERIES EDITORS
Graeme Duthie MD, FRCS(Ed), FRCS
and
Diane Palmer BSc(Hons), RN, PGCE

W

WHURR PUBLISHERS
LONDON AND PHILADELPHIA

© 2004 Whurr Publishers

First Published 2004
Whurr Publishers Ltd
19b Compton Terrace, London N1 2UN, England and
325 Chestnut Street, Philadelphia PA19106, USA

British Library Cataloguing in Publication Data

A catalogue record for this book is available from the
British Library.

ISBN 1 86156 265 9

Printed and bound in the UK by Athenaeum Press Limited,
Gateshead, Tyne & Wear.

Contents

Contributors

Liz Ashton, MBChB, MRCPsych, *Consultant Psychiatrist, Ellis Centre, Scarborough, UK*

Pamela Barker, RGN *Nutrition Nurse Specialist, Scarborough Hospital, Scarborough, UK*

Mandie Bulmer RGN, BSc(Hons), *Nurse Practitioner, Castle Hill Hospital, East Yorkshire Hospitals NHS Trust, Hull, UK*

S. Robin Cohen, PhD, *Research Director and Assistant Professor, Division of Palliative Care, Department of Oncology, McGill University and Medical Scientist, Department of Medicine, McGill University Health Centre, Montreal, Canada*

Sue Davis, RN, BN, MN, *Clinical Nurse Consultant, Palliative Care, Sir Charles Gairdner Hospital, Perth, Western Australia*

Graeme Duthie, MD, FRCS(Ed), FRCS, *Consultant GI Surgeon, Castle Hill Hospital, Hull and East Yorkshire Hospitals NHS Trust, Hull, UK*

Linda J. Kristjanson, RN, BN, MN, PhD, *Professor, School of Nursing and Public Health, Associate Dean (Research and Higher Degrees), Faculty of Communications, Health and Science, Edith Cowan University, Churchlands, Western Australia*

Sally Legge, RGN, MSc, Onc Cert, *Clinical Nurse Specialist, Gastro-Intestinal-Unit, Royal Marsden NHS Trust, London, UK*

Tracey McCready, RGN, BSc, HETC, ICTM, *Tutor in Nursing, University of Hull, Hull, UK*

Julie MacDonald, MSc (Palliative Care), RGN, BSc, RM, Cert Ed, ILTM, *Tutor in Nursing, University of Hull, Hull, UK*

Suzanne Nikoletti, PhD, RN, *Senior Lecturer, School of Nursing and Public Health, Edith Cowan University, Director, Nursing Practice Research Network, Sir Charles Gairdner Hospital, and Research Consultant, Cancer Nursing Research Network, Sir Charles Gairdner Hospital, Perth, Western Australia*

Diane Palmer, BSc(Hons), RN, PGCE *Lecturer in Nursing, University of Hull, Hull, UK*

Davina Porock, PhD, RN, *Associate Professor, Sinclair School of Nursing, University of Missouri-Columbia, Missouri, USA*

Fran Rhys Evans, MSc, RN, Onc Cert, *Department of Head and Neck Surgery, Royal Marsden NHS Trust, London, UK*

Peter Rhys Evans, MBBS, LRCP, FRCS, DCC, *Consultant, Department of Head and Neck Surgery, Royal Marsden NHS Trust, London, UK*

Peter Sedman, FRCS, *Consultant Surgeon, Department of General Surgery, Hull and East Yorkshire Hospitals NHS Trust, Hull, UK*

Hanif Shiwani, FRCSI, *Consultant Surgeon, Barnsley District Hospital, South Yorkshire, UK*

Karen Tarhuni, RGN, *Senior Nurse, Department of General Surgery, Hull and East Yorkshire Hospitals NHS Trust, Hull, UK*

Series Foreword

This series represents a significant addition to the nursing literature. The editors are respected experts and they have assembled a team of authors with the necessary experience and reputation to ensure the authority of each volume. From the stable of the prestigious specialist nurse endoscopy course at the University of Hull and based in the Hull and East Yorkshire Hospitals NHS Trust, this series will ensure that excellence will not be the preserve of these institutions.

Gastroenterology is an important field where nurses can develop and practise as specialist and advanced practitioners. The field extends from the inexplicable, such as irritable bowel syndrome, through the aetiological puzzle of inflammatory bowel disease, to life-threatening malignancies. Irritable bowel syndrome and inflammatory bowel disease both involve significant psychological morbidity and treatment in these areas is ripe for the development of nursing interventions such as counselling and behavioural therapies. Definitive diagnosis of inflammatory disorders and malignancies requires endoscopy, and this is an area where nursing makes a significant contribution through independent practice. Endoscopy is an invasive procedure which raises significant anxiety in patients and one where nurses are able to combine their psychosocial and technical skills. As such, nurses require well developed psychosocial skills – which are integral to nursing practice – and a deep knowledge of the anatomy and physiology of the gastrointestinal tract. The series will ensure that all nurses, particularly those who wish to practise in the field of gastroenterology, will have a sound foundation.

Roger Watson BSc, PhD, RGN, CBiol, FIBiol, ILTM, FRSA
Professor of Nursing, University of Hull

Preface

The care of the patient with cancer is a demanding but satisfying specialty in nursing. Contemporary oncology nursing practice relies on a broad knowledge base from the biomedical and behavioural sciences. Understanding the patient as an individual within the context of the family, work and environment is as important to the oncology nurse as knowledge of cancer as a disease and its treatment. Cancer is often referred to as a journey. Oncology nurses become part of the cancer journey as the patient travels from diagnosis and treatment to survival or death. This book focuses on the nursing care of the patient with cancer of the gastrointestinal tract and is intended as a primer for nurses who may not have experience in the oncology specialty.

The book begins with a comprehensive examination of the issues and scope of the frequently used term 'quality of life', providing a thorough critique of its meaning and assessment in practice. This content is presented as the first chapter because promotion of quality of life for the patient and family is a major concern of oncology nursing practice. To be effective the nurse needs a clear understanding of quality of life, how to measure it and how to evaluate the impact of nursing interventions. Chapters 2 and 3 take an in-depth look at the impact of cancer on the individual and the family. The purpose of these two chapters is to consider the cancer patient as an individual within the context of the family, providing practical suggestions for understanding and helping the patient and family. These three chapters form the foundation for the subsequent chapters.

Chapters 4-6 introduce the principal aspects of cancer as a disease from both a medical and a nursing perspective, beginning with cancers of the aerodigestive tract through to lower gastrointestinal cancers. Each chapter is written by medical and nurse co-authors to provide a more complete view of patient care. Chapter 7 covers the role of nutrition in the prevention of cancer and the nutritional management of patients with cancer.

The final three chapters of the book focus on the specific nursing care of the patient undergoing cancer treatment. Chapters 8 and 9 provide a guide to the management of patients undergoing radiotherapy and chemotherapy in order to familiarize the gastroenterology nurse with what may lie ahead for the patient. The chapters are not designed to prepare the nurse to administer chemotherapy or work in the specialty of radiotherapy, but rather to become aware of the major issues and the experience of patients. The final chapter outlines the principles of symptom management and palliative care for integration into patient care throughout the cancer journey.

Cancer of the Gastrointestinal Tract: A handbook for nurse practitioners is one of a series of texts written for the gastroenterology nurse. The book does not include information on cancer at a cellular level; the reader is directed to the many comprehensive texts that are already available. The aim here is to provide a sufficiently broad introduction and discussion of oncology nursing with a clear focus on patient- and family-centred care.

Davina Porock and Diane Palmer
November 2003

CHAPTER 1

Quality of life and the cancer journey

SUZANNE NIKOLETTI AND ROBIN COHEN

A diagnosis of cancer has a profound impact on the quality of life of patients and their families. This chapter traces the theoretical underpinnings of quality of life in relation to cancer. The aim is to provide a context for subsequent chapters in which the events, treatment options and management strategies can be considered more readily from the patient's perspective. Although the quality of life of family members is important as well, it is not covered in this chapter.

Why should we study quality of life?

Patients engage the healthcare system because they have suffering that needs to be relieved (Mechanic, 1962). For those with cancer, anticancer treatment may relieve part of the suffering, but the diagnosis and treatment both produce suffering that is not addressed by interventions focusing on the body alone. Quality of life – a person's subjective sense of well-being – has become an important area of cancer research in the last few decades. The impetus for much of this research can be linked to significant advances in medical technology and cancer treatments, which have resulted in prolonged survival times for many patients. Such treatments, while increasing the quantity of life, are often aggressive and may cause severe side effects, which compromise quality of life. Furthermore, in situations where cancer treatments are non-curative and aim instead to improve comfort or function, quality rather than quantity of life becomes the central concern for patients and their families. In addition, the diagnosis of a life-threatening illness such as cancer has itself a tremendous impact on quality of life, not only in negative ways, but also in some positive ways.

The importance of measuring quality of life has been well documented (de Haes and van Knippenberg, 1985; Aaronson, 1990; King et al., 1997). 'Quality of life studies and measurements serve to prevent a devastating separation of a patient's body from a patient's biography during delivery of care' (Roy, 1992, p. 4). From a theoretical perspective, studies on quality of life help us to understand the effect of cancer and cancer treatments on patients. The results of such research can influence decisions about choice of therapy, e.g. if two treatments have the same impact on survival, but one leads to a better quality of life, or if one gives better survival at the expense of quality of life, patients can make an informed decision. Knowledge gained by health professionals can be used to monitor the quality of care and enhance supportive care, through specific interventions. Individual patients can be screened for the need for interventions that may otherwise be overlooked, particularly in relation to psychosocial and spiritual well-being. Quality-of-life studies can inform us about the effectiveness of the communication of health professionals with patients. Finally, efforts can be directed towards developing preventive measures that support adjustment and minimize complications.

Evaluating the trade-off between quality and quantity of life in the face of aggressive treatments is a difficult task, even for qualified health professionals, e.g. the arguments for and against aggressive treatments for patients with advanced colorectal cancer have recently been debated by experts in the field (Blijham et al., 1997; Redmond, 1998a, 1998b). Such debates are complicated by the differing perspectives held by patients and health professionals on what patients could be expected to tolerate. A number of studies have revealed that patients, on average, are likely to choose more aggressive treatments than healthy observers state that they themselves would tolerate (Bremnes et al., 1995). However, the choice of individual patients will vary. Therefore, it is important that patients are included in the decision-making process and that they have access to the results of quality-of-life research to guide their choice of treatment.

Finally, some may benefit from participation in quality-of-life research (Cohen et al., 1995; Ferrell, 1996). Patients appreciate the opportunity to articulate important aspects of their lives that may have been overlooked in their treatment to date. Patients appear to benefit by gaining a new perspective on their lives or by having their feelings validated by others.

Quality of life: emerging trends

Since the 1970s, there has been growing interest in the study of quality of life associated with diseases such as cancer and their associated treatments. Before the 1990s, most studies on quality of life suffered from the use of instruments or checklists that measured limited aspects or antecedents of quality of life, such as physical functioning or symptoms, rather than instruments based on theoretically derived models of quality of life (Bowling, 1995). In the last decade, however, the recognition of quality of life as a multidimensional phenomenon has resulted in the development of quality-of-life instruments that measure a broader range of domains, including at least physical, psychological and social well-being, with a more recent trend to include spiritual well-being and other domains as well. Some of these instruments, such as the European Organisation for Research and Treatment of Cancer Quality of Life Questionnaire (EORTC-QLQ – Aaronson et al., 1993) and the Functional Assessment of Cancer Therapy (FACT – Cella et al., 1993), have been developed as core measures, supplemented by disease site- or treatment-specific modules that can provide more detail about concerns specific to a particular type of cancer or treatment. These are discussed in more detail in relation to the measurement of quality of life.

Another important trend emerging in the last decade has been the move away from health professionals' ratings of patients' quality of life to the use of patient self-reports. Many researchers now regard the subjectivity of patients' evaluations of quality of life as a strength rather than a limitation, and have promoted the use of qualitative approaches to gain insights into the defining elements of quality of life from patients' perspectives (Padilla et al., 1990; King et al., 1997). However, there has been only limited research on theoretical foundations of quality of life. Consequently, our understanding of the essence of quality of life is still in its early stages, despite the existence of numerous operational definitions of this phenomenon.

What is quality of life?

Understanding the defining elements or conceptual domains of quality of life is important in helping nurses understand what is important to cancer patients and their families. Some aspects of the cancer journey that need to be considered include the emotional and practical impact of diagnosis, disease effects, decision-making, treatments, and short- and long-term side effects, financial concerns, environment, prognosis, terminal illness, and fears about pain, loss, grief and the future. Specific concerns relating to patients with different diagnoses are discussed in subsequent chapters. This section focuses on describing the theoretical foundations of quality of life that apply to all stages of the cancer journey, even though the relative importance of specific domains of quality of life may vary along the health and illness continuum and from individual to individual.

There have been many attempts to formulate a consensus definition of quality of life. Donovan et al. (1989) state that a generally agreed definition is 'a person's subjective sense of well-being derived from current experience of life as a whole'. Cantril (1965) studied satisfaction with life and found it to be determined by the discrepancy between the life that we want to have and the life that we perceive ourselves to have. Others have produced evidence supporting this hypothesis (Campbell et al., 1976; Najman and Levine, 1981). More recently, Calman (1984) has applied this to quality of life, suggesting that it reflects the difference or gap between the hopes and expectations of a person and the present experience. Some researchers have proposed that healthcare workers should ignore the broader implications of quality of life and focus instead on that part of quality of life that is directly related to health care – referring to 'health-related quality of life,' defined as that which 'refers to the extent to which one's usual or expected physical, emotional, and social well-being are affected by a medical condition or its treatment' (Cella, 1995). This definition does not include such factors as housing, income and perceptions of immediate environment (Bowling, 1995). Nor, according to Aaronson (1990), should it include such general issues as happiness and life satisfaction because these are claimed to be 'so distal to the goals and objectives of health care that it would seem inappropriate to apply them as criteria against which to judge the efficacy of medical interventions'. This narrower view of quality of life runs counter to the philosophy that underpins holistic nursing care. Moreover, it seems to ignore the evidence that quality of life is determined by the *interaction* between each individual and the objective situation at a given time (Gill and Feinstein, 1994; Mount and Cohen, 1995). Thus, a diagnosis of cancer and the effects of treatment will be evaluated in many different ways according to who we are and not simply by what is happening to us medically.

The following discussion expands on four important aspects of quality of life: its subjectivity, dynamism (Allison et al., 1997), multidimensionality (Cella, 1994), and positive and negative dimensions (Calman, 1984; Donovan et al., 1989; Cohen and Mount, 1992; Hyland, 1992; Bowling, 1995, p. 2).

Subjectivity and dynamism

One way of expressing the subjective nature of quality of life (QoL) is that it is whatever the patient says it is – a definition frequently used for pain. In other words, QoL can be understood only from the patient's perspective (Cohen and Mount, 1992; Cella, 1994). As quality of life is a perception, it is dynamic in nature and will change for a given person over time, even in the same objective situation (Mount and Cohen, 1995; Allison et al., 1997). These two aspects of quality of life are closely related and are discussed together.

There is often a discrepancy among patient self-reports of quality of life, observers' ratings of a patient's quality of life and objective clinical indicators such as physical deterioration and survival, e.g. Cassileth et al. (1982) found the psychological well-being of a group of melanoma patients to be significantly better than that of a group of patients with other dermatological disorders and slightly better than that of a sample of the general population. In addition, discrepancies between patient self-reports of quality of life and ratings of patient quality of life by others are common (de Haes and van Knippenberg, 1985; Breetvelt and Van Dam, 1991; Cohen and Mount, 1992; Sprangers and Aaronson, 1992; Bowling, 1995; Allison et al., 1997). The discrepancy between subjective and objective measures is explained partly by the fact that they are not measuring exactly the same thing (Allison et al., 1997). However, the discrepancies between patient self-reports and observers' expectations point to the essentially subjective nature of quality of life. Patients often rate their quality of life more highly than observers do, particularly in situations such as terminal illness. Obviously, the patients perceive some strong positive contributors to quality of life, in the face of extreme physical decline and impending death.

What is the impact of the subjective and dynamic nature of quality-of-life evaluations? If a person's external environment is changing, while the self-reported evaluation of well-being remains fairly constant, then the person must be altering his or her internal standards to accommodate the change. Allison et al. (1997) have reviewed a large body of literature that provides evidence for the psychological processes contributing to these changing internal standards. These and other processes that have been proposed to explain the subjective nature of quality of life are summarized in Table 1.1.

Given the number of psychological factors that may influence an individual's perception of quality of life, it is not surprising that the point of reference for evaluating quality of life differs from person to person. However, the potential for this point of reference to change for each individual over time must also be considered. The growing evidence that people continue to rate their quality of life as acceptable, even in what are objectively difficult circumstances (Cassileth et al., 1982; Decker and Schultz, 1985; Evans, 1991; Cohen and Mount, 1992), supports Maslow's (1954, p. 24) contention that people's expectations are usually within the realm of the possible. The degree of life satisfaction, happiness or quality of life perceived is found in the discrepancy between people's perceptions of their current situation and their expectations (Cantril, 1965; Campbell et al., 1976; Calman, 1984). Kreitler and colleagues (1993) hypothesize that the changing criteria used by an individual to judge his or her own situation are a necessary adaptation that humans have developed to ward off debilitating depression. According to Golembiewski et al. (1976), this 'within-subject' change, or dynamism, can be at two levels, referred to as beta and gamma.

In the case of beta change, there is a shift or recalibration within the measurement continuum. Thus, one's perception of the worst pain imaginable may change after having endured severe pain at a level far worse than any previously experienced (Allison et al., 1997).

Gamma change involves a redefinition of what is being measured, e.g. a healthy person may state that the important

Table 1.1 Psychological constructs that may explain the subjective and dynamic nature of quality of life

Construct	Brief outline
1. Adaptation	The individual's achievement of an acceptable level of well-being through the meanings that are given to past, present and future situations (Heyink, 1993) (based on Helson's [1964] adaptation theory)
2. Coping	A similar concept to adaptation, but emphasizes stressors and the individual's attempts to deal with them (Lazarus and Folkman, 1984). An individual's coping resources are complex and involve personal, social, and material factors. Furthermore, coping resources may change according to the stressor
3. Control theory of self-awareness	When individuals focus attention on themselves, they compare their current state with important goals and values. If the gap between reality and these goals and values is too large, behavioural adjustments are made to move closer to these desired states (Carver and Scheier, 1982)
4. Self-concept	Includes self-esteem. Refers to how people feel about themselves in terms of physical, psychosocial, achievement and spiritual domains (Foltz, 1987)
5. Expectancy	The belief that a certain action will result in a certain outcome (Scheier and Carver, 1987). The placebo effect is one of the best examples of the effect of expectancies on subjective health (Allison et al., 1997)
6. Self-efficacy	Related to expectancy, but refers to an individual's belief that he or she has the ability to perform an action that achieves an outcome (Bandura, 1982)
7. Optimism	A stable personality characteristic that affects expectancies, behaviour and health (Scheier and Carver, 1985), and is associated with a higher level of well-being (Scheier and Carver, 1987)
8. Uncertainty	May be valued by an individual as positive, offering hope (opportunity), or negative (danger). People with progressively deteriorating illness appear to evaluate uncertainty associated with the illness and treatment more positively than healthy people or health professionals (Mishel, 1988)
9. Affect	The emotional response to an experience, more strongly related to physical status and sensitive to short-term change (de Haes and van Knippenberg, 1985)
10. Cognition	The rational appraisal of an experience (reasoning, thinking, satisfaction), more strongly related to personality and thus more stable than affect over the short term (de Haes and van Knippenberg, 1985)

(contd)

Table 1.1 (contd)

Construct	Brief outline
11. Problem/ Evaluation	In this conceptualization of quality-of-life measurement, problems refer to a person's cognitive knowledge of health status, determined by the presence of symptoms. Evaluation refers to the personal appraisal of health status and involves psychological factors (Hyland, 1992). These constructs are related to the cognitive/affective constructs described above, but problem items are reported to be more sensitive to change (long term) over time (Hyland et al., 1994)
12. Denial	Based on the psychoanalytic theory of 'defence mechanisms' whereby the patient denies the threatening reality, preventing it from entering the conscious realm (Breetvelt and Van Dam, 1991)
13. Downward social comparison	Cancer patients' tendency to compare themselves with others who are worse off, thus changing their internal standards for evaluating quality of life (Breetvelt and Van Dam, 1991) (based on social Comparison Theory [Festinger, 1954])
14. Discrepancy theories and cognitive flexibility	Better quality of life occurs when patients' experiences match their expectations (Linder-Petz, 1982). People who are more cognitively flexible are able to modify their expectations of quality of life under deteriorating circumstances and are therefore likely to rate their quality of life higher than someone with similar problems who is less adaptable (Cella, 1994)
15. Maslow's hierarchy of needs theory and adaptation theory	Maslow (1954) suggested that human needs exist in a hierarchy such that basic needs (e.g. physiological, safety) must be satisfied before an individual can work on higher level needs (e.g. self-esteem and self-actualization). Maslow also noted that human adaptation is such that life expectations are usually adjusted to lie within the realm of what the individual perceives to be possible

quality of life factors for him or her are health, family, work and financial status. However, after diagnosis and treatment of life-threatening cancer, new quality-of-life domains, such as spiritual well-being, may be identified by the same person. In addition, specific contributors to quality of life may change or have increased or decreased importance, e.g. health for someone with cancer of the head/neck region or the gastrointestinal tract may be redefined as ability to talk, eat or have normal bowel function (Allison et al., 1997). Other contributors, such as work attainment or financial goals, may no longer be important for some people, whereas for others they may become more important, representing indicators of the return to a normal and fulfilling life.

Evidence for gamma change comes from the work of Kreitler et al. (1993), who demonstrated that head and neck cancer patients had a similar degree of life satisfaction to orthopaedic patients and physically healthy people. However, the cancer patients derived their life satisfaction from many more domains than the other individuals (ten vs three domains). Furthermore, the domains related to health had a decreased contribution to the life satisfaction of the cancer patients compared with the other individuals, although the domains not related to health (work, economic state, family life, parenthood, communication with partner, sexuality, getting help, social life and entertainment) made a relatively increased contribution.

In summary, cancer patients' capacity for adaptation means that they may rate their quality of life more highly than do observers such as family or health professionals. In addition, patients may be more tolerant of the effects of disease or aggressive treatments. The dynamic nature of these subjective evaluations adds further complexity to the assessment and interpretation of cancer patients' quality of life over the disease trajectory. However, if quality of life is defined as subjective well-being, shifts in the reference point by which quality of life is judged should be viewed as an integral part of the perception of quality of life, rather than as a bothersome problem in quality-of-life measurement (Sprangers, 1996). On the other hand, if we are interested in measuring the impact of a specific intervention on a specific symptom or set of symptoms, these are best measured directly rather than measuring quality of life, and perhaps people should be asked directly to rate changes in these symptoms.

Multidimensionality of quality of life

If we accept that a good definition of quality of life is 'subjective well-being' (Mount and Cohen, 1995), we need to determine the dimensions or core domains that contribute to this phenomenon. Although there is still no consensus among researchers (King et al., 1997), at least five key domains can be identified from the literature – physical, functional, emotional (psychological), social and spiritual well-being (Padilla et al., 1990; Cohen and Mount, 1992; Cella, 1994; Ferrell et al., 1995b; Cohen et al., 1996; King et al., 1997). Interviews with patients with advanced cancer also suggest that communication and access to information are important domains, along with cognitive functioning (Cohen, 2003a, 2003b). These domains are listed in Table 1.2, along with examples of items related to each domain.

It should be noted, however, that there is considerable variation in the number and types of domains that are included within different quality-of-life instruments. In addition, the relative emphasis given to items within each domain may vary, e.g. some instruments do not include spiritual well-being and others have a greater proportion of items within the physical and functional domains. In some conceptual frameworks, the physical and functional domains are combined (Ferrell et al., 1995b).

Other differences worth noting are that similar domains may be labelled differently among researchers, and there is some variability in the distribution of items across the domains, reflecting their inter-relatedness, e.g. sexuality can be expressed through, and is influenced by, physical, functional, emotional and social domains (Cella, 1994). Similarly, there is some overlap in the distribution of items within functional and social domains, functional and physical domains, or psychological and spiritual or existential domains.

Within the physical domain, the distinction between disease and treatment effects may become blurred to the patient, who may view these experiences as an aggregate, or misinterpret symptoms as side effects, or vice versa (Cella, 1994). Functional well-being is correlated with, but considered by Cella (1994) to be conceptually distinct from, physical well-being. It refers to the ability to perform the activities related to personal needs, ambitions or one's social role. Psychological well-being has two separate dimensions, reflecting positive affect (well-being) as well as negative affect (distress). These are separate rather than two ends of a continuum (Bradburn, 1969). Social well-being is a poorly understood dimension and not thoroughly addressed in most scales (Cella, 1994). The fifth domain, spirituality, is another dimension that has not been adequately addressed in most quality-of-life studies. It is recognized by nurses to be central to quality of life and holistic nursing care (Belcher et al., 1989; O'Connor et al., 1990; Ferrell et al., 1992a; Grant et al.,

Table 1.2 Core domains of quality of life

Core domains	Examples of items (not comprehensive)
Physical	Disease symptoms Treatment side effects, e.g. nausea, appetite and weight changes, pain, fatigue and disfigurement

Functional	Capacity for activities relating to:
	    daily living (self care)
	    work
	    hobbies
	    school
	    fulfilment of responsibilities to family,
	    friends and work colleagues
	ability to access information
	ability to communicate

Psychological	Anxiety Depression Anger Other emotional distress Self-esteem Internal locus of control Happiness Optimism Joy Contentment Body image Uncertainty
Social	Leisure activities Isolation Social support Family functioning Intimacy Sexual relations
Spiritual/Existential	Strengthened belief Usefulness Being fulfilled Satisfaction with life Hope Religiosity Inner strength Meaning of illness Spirituality Transcendence Control Uncertainty

From Padilla et al. (1990), Cohen and Mount (1992), Cella (1994), Ferrell et al. (1995b), Cohen et al. (1996), King et al. (1997) and Cohen (2003a).

1992; Highfield, 1992; Fryback, 1993; Kahn and Steeves, 1993; Coward, 1994; King et al., 1997).

Evidence from other disciplines on the importance of the spiritual and existential domain comes from studies of patients with cancer or AIDS and in terminally ill individuals (Cohen and Mount, 1996; Cohen et al., 1996; Cohen et al., 1997b; Brady et al., 1999). Part of the problem underlying the lack of acceptance of spirituality may relate to the misconception that it concerns only religious associations. However, as shown in Table 1.2, items within this domain encompass far more than religiosity. Indeed, spiritual well-being does not necessarily include any formal religious practice or affiliation (Cohen and Mount, 1992; Ferrell et al., 1995b). Nevertheless, the incorporation of this domain within a health-related quality-of-life model is still not universally supported, with some researchers arguing for its exclusion on the questionable grounds that such issues lie outside the goals of health care (Aaronson, 1990). However, as quality of life is a perception (subjective) of the person, all aspects of that person are relevant to and will affect their rating of quality of life, not only those on which the healthcare system focuses. Furthermore, existential concerns increase after a cancer diagnosis and so are important to the patients (Weisman and Worden, 1976; Gotay, 1985; Belcher et al., 1989; Fryback, 1993).

If quality of life is subjective well-being, then we must measure the perceived *effect* of specific contributors to quality of life, rather than the degree to which these specific contributors are present, e.g. physical symptoms will contribute to quality of life, but the extent of that contribution will depend on many factors. To give a concrete example, one person with moderate hip pain may find it greatly affects her quality of life because it makes it difficult to get to the only toilet in the house, which is upstairs. Another may find the same pain has much less impact on quality of life because she has a toilet on each floor! Therefore, if quality of life, rather than the symptoms, is of interest, it is important to measure the *impact* of the symptom rather than its intensity. If, however, the symptoms themselves are of interest, a symptom assessment tool rather than a quality-of-life instrument should be used.

It has been suggested that neither a single definition nor a single quality-of-life scale will adequately capture changes in quality of life at all points along the continuum of cancer care

(Bowling, 1995; King et al., 1997). Factors that need to be considered include disease status, treatment point (pre-, during, post-), or primary location of care (home, hospital). Future studies will need to determine which instruments function best in each set of circumstances, and whether there is an instrument that will be useful in all circumstances.

Positive and negative dimensions of quality of life

Evidence for positive and negative contributors to psychological well-being comes from Bradburn's (1969) large study which shows that the amount of negative affect people feel is not related to the amount of positive affect they feel. Further evidence of the lack of correlation between positive and negative determinants of well-being is revealed in the work of Costa and McCrae (1980) on life satisfaction, and that of Watson and Pennebaker (1989) on mood. These studies suggest that the positive and negative determinants exert their effects through different causal processes, and therefore the two constructs should be measured separately. For the same reasons, nurses in clinical settings should consider the need to address both positive determinants (e.g. happiness, contentment, optimism, inner strength, usefulness) and negative determinants (disease and treatment effects, anxiety, depression, anger) of quality of life when assessing patients and planning for their care.

The work of nurse researchers has also revealed the importance of positive contributors to quality of life (Fryback, 1993; Kagawa-Singer, 1993; Ferrell, 1996). Studies of quality of life in long-term cancer survivors have identified several strengths gained from the cancer experience, including hopefulness, having a purpose in life, improving personal relationships, feeling useful, and having a deeper sense of life and joy (Ferrell et al., 1995b). Thus, there is considerable evidence that the absence of health problems will not result in a high quality of life without positive contributions in other domains. On the other hand, even severe illness may be associated with good quality of life as a result of positive contributors (Mount and Cohen, 1995; Cohen and Mount, 1996; Cohen et al., 1996, 1997a). Unfortunately, most instruments in current use focus almost entirely on the negative aspects associated with the disease. In clinical practice, the tendency to focus on dealing with problems may result in the neglect of opportunities to build on patients' strengths and positive capacities.

How should quality of life be measured?

To answer this question, first we must know the purpose for which the measurement is intended. Researchers aiming to study quality of life as an outcome of cancer or cancer treatment for a population will have different needs to clinicians who may want to assess aspects of quality of life to guide individual patient care. Most quality-of-life instruments available at present have been designed for research purposes and their scores may not be appropriate for clinical use without further amendments. However, instruments designed purely for research can be useful in a clinical context, as a means of promoting communication about issues that might otherwise go unmentioned.

Another important question would be to ask what nurses would do with the information gained from quality-of-life assessments. Without the commitment to use the information to guide practice, collecting quality-of-life data routinely in the clinical setting becomes a meaningless task. Recent studies have shown that nurses (Eischens et al., 1998) and physicians (Pratheepawanit et al., 1999) find standardized instruments useful in guiding treatment for individual patients, especially in complex cases (Pratheepawanit et al., 1999).

Types of quality-of-life instruments

In broad terms, quality-of-life instruments can be divided into five main groups: (1) generic measures; (2) single-item or global measures; (3) disease- or treatment-specific measures; (4) domain-specific measures; and (5) individualized measures. Each of these is discussed below.

Generic measures

Generic instruments such as the World Health Organization Quality of Life Assessment (World Health Organization, 1998) can be used to measure quality of life in physically healthy populations, as well as in those with all types of physical illness. These are useful when there is a need to compare quality of life across populations (e.g. to compare the quality-of-life of people with diabetes or cancer with that of the general population). Generic instruments are important, but are not discussed further in this chapter, which focuses on cancer-specific measures.

Single-item (global) measures

An example of a single-item measure is the question 'How would you rate your quality of life today?'. Gough et al. (1983) suggest that only a single question of this type is required to evaluate quality of life of patients with advanced cancer. This recommendation is supported by the demonstration of strong correlations between scores on single-item and multi-item scales (Gough et al., 1983; Sloan et al., 1998).

Gill and Feinstein (1994) also promote the use of single global ratings. However, they recommend two separate measures, one for overall quality of life and one for health-related quality of life, to determine the impact of so-called non-medical phenomena such as employment, family relationships and spirituality. The practical value of such a distinction is debatable, given the recognized conceptual links among health, social support and spiritual well-being in nursing models of care (Neuman, 1974) and in definitions of 'health' given by cancer patients (Fryback, 1993; Kagawa-Singer, 1993).

Single-item scales are useful and appear to be valid for certain research purposes when an overall quality-of-life measure is required, e.g. in exploratory or hypothesis-generating studies (Sloan et al., 1998). Sloan et al. (1998) recommend the use of a single-item scale when measuring overall changes over time, because they found the single-item scale had greater sensitivity to change compared with a multi-item tool. This is because for a change to appear numerically on a single-item scale only a single response is needed. However, to see a substantive change of quality of life using a multi-item scale, responses in a number of components have to change and the effect of some changes can be cancelled out if negative changes (such as loss of mobility and independence) balance the positive changes (such as improved relationships with family). This apparent advantage must be weighed against the likelihood that the stability (test–retest reliability) of single-item scales is often low. This arises because errors may tend to be mainly in a single direction for a given item. The effect of this tendency is usually less in multi-item scales because different items have errors in different directions, with the average error tending towards zero. If the scale does not have acceptable test–retest reliability, it will be difficult to detect real change, i.e. change that is not the result of error (Streiner and Norman, 1995).

In summary, the decision to use a single-item versus a multi-item tool should be guided by the purpose of the study – the use of both is often the best option. The single-item tool offers the advantage of reflecting more accurately what the patient means by quality of life. Multi-item tools offer benefits when assessment of more specific information is required to understand, interpret or act on a global rating. In the clinical setting, it is unlikely that a questionnaire could ever replace a good clinical interview. However, individual items or domains within multi-item tools may serve as useful checkpoints or indicators, upon which more detailed assessment and subsequent care and evaluation can be based. The systematic documentation of information about multiple areas of concern may help the nurse to identify priorities for individual patients, using questions such as 'What is most important for you right now?'.

Specific measures

Disease- or situation-specific measures

Disease- or situation-specific instruments for cancer populations are multi-item tools that measure well-being across a number of domains relevant to all types of cancer. Sometimes they are created as 'core' measures, relevant to all types of cancer, with cancer site-specific 'modules' or versions that add items relevant to specific types of cancer. The EORTC QLQ-C30 series is one example (Aaronson et al., 1993). It consists of 30 items that measure physical, mental, psychological, social and financial status, as well as global quality of life. It may be supplemented by site- or treatment-specific modules. Although the EORTC series is the most widely used quality-of-life measure in oncology, it suffers from having been developed from the perspectives of oncologists, rather than from the perspectives of patients. In addition, its overemphasis on the physical domain makes this instrument inappropriate for patients with advanced cancer.

Another well-established system is the FACT series (Cella et al., 1993), which consists of a core instrument, the FACT–General (FACT-G), and site-specific modules for a wide range of conditions. The FACT-G produces subscale scores for physical, functional, social and emotional well-being, as well as satisfaction with the treatment relationship.

Other instruments have been developed to measure the quality of life of cancer patients that do not have site- or treatment-specific modules. One of these is the Spitzer Quality of Life Index (Spitzer et al., 1981). It can be rated by staff or patients, and has five items concerning activity, activities of daily living, overall health, outlook and support. The Functional Living Index–Cancer (FLIC) (Schipper et al., 1984) measures physical and occupational functioning, psychological state, sociability and somatic comfort. These two questionnaires give a measure of overall quality of life. The McGill Quality of Life Questionnaire (Cohen and Mount, 1996; Cohen et al., 1996, 1997b) is a situation-specific instrument designed for patients with life-threatening illness of any type. It includes a single-item measure of quality of life, a summary measure of overall quality of life, and subscale scores measuring physical symptoms, physical well-being, psychological symptoms, existential well-being and support.

The Quality of Life Index of Ferrans and Powers (1985) was first tested with haemodialysis patients and later modified for cancer patients (Ferrans, 1990). It covers a broad range of domains, including physical, functional, psychological, family, social, economic and spiritual/existential. Patients are asked to rate their satisfaction for each item, as well as its importance, and a weighted score is calculated. The Quality of Life–Cancer Survivors (QOL-CS) (Ferrell et al., 1995a, 1995b) is based on several previous instruments (Ferrell et al., 1989, 1992a, 1992b; Padilla et al., 1990; Grant et al., 1992). The revised version includes issues of concern for cancer survivors (identified through in-depth qualitative interviews) and has items representing the psychological, physical, social and spiritual domains. The McMaster Quality of Life Scale (Sterkenburg, 1996), the Missoula-VITAS Quality of Life Index (Byock and Merriman, 1998) and the Hospice Quality of Life Index (McMillan and Mahon, 1994) were developed specifically for the palliative phase, but might be useful at earlier phases as well, although this remains to be tested.

Site- or treatment-specific measures

Patients with cancers affecting different body sites experience a variety of disease and treatment side effects that impact on quality of life in different ways and to different degrees. Therefore, for some purposes, the core measures described above may not adequately assess the effect of a specific disease or treatment on quality of life, e.g. a study of quality of life in oesophageal cancer patients receiving two different types of treatment (oesophagectomy vs palliation) found that dysphagia, the most predominant symptom, did not significantly correlate with any of the items, or with any of the functional or symptom scales on the EORTC core questionnaire (Blazeby et al., 1995). This finding indicates the need to supplement the core questionnaire with a site-specific module that will more specifically measure some of the anticipated effects of an intervention if these, rather than overall quality of life or quality of life in specific domains, are of primary interest. An awareness of this need across a variety of site-specific cancers has led researchers to develop site- or treatment-specific quality-of-life measures that are sensitive to small, but clinically significant changes.

Site- or treatment-specific quality-of-life indicators are generally designed to be supplemented with a generic or core measure. The EORTC QLQ series is one example of this approach. Sprangers et al. (1998) provide an overview of the 16 modules of the EORTC series currently under development or available, including those for colorectal, head and neck, pancreatic and oesophageal cancer, as well as for high-dose chemotherapy and body image. Studies of the psychometric properties of the modules for colorectal cancer (Sprangers et al., 1999) and head and neck cancer (Bjordal et al., 1999) have recently been published. The EORTC modules are used in conjunction with the core instrument, the EORTC QLQ-C30, which has been translated into many different languages and is now being widely used in clinical trials throughout Europe, Canada, the USA and Australia.

The Functional Assessment of Chronic Illness Therapy (FACIT) measurement system is another well-established group of instruments, including a core measure, the FACT (Cella et al., 1993), and a range of site-specific modules. Those relevant to gastrointestinal cancer include the FACT-HNS for head and neck cancer (List et al., 1996), the FACT-C for colorectal cancer (Ward et al., 1999), the FACT-F for fatigue and the FACT-An for anaemia (Yellen et al., 1997).

Padilla and colleagues have developed a visual analogue scale for patients with colostomies (Quality of Life Index–Colostomy) (Padilla and Grant, 1985). This scale is a site-specific extension of the Quality of Life Index (Padilla et al., 1983), later renamed the Multidimensional Quality of Life Scale–Cancer (Padilla et al., 1992).

Despite the widespread use of the EORTC modules, no single instrument has been identified as the gold standard, reflecting the lack of agreement about what should be measured and the different contexts in which quality of life is studied. In fact, Aaronson (1990) argues that there is a danger in elevating a single instrument to gold standard status, and that the pursuit of such a goal is misguided, because no instrument is perfect in all situations. Furthermore, a 'gold standard' label can seriously hamper attempts to improve the instrument, an opinion shared by King et al. (1997) who predict the continuing evolution of the conceptual definition of quality of life, and consequently the need to integrate this new knowledge into our assessment tools on an ongoing basis.

Domain-specific measures

Domain-specific instruments measure only specific aspects of, or contributors to, quality of life, rather than quality of life itself. Bowling (1995, pp. 24–27) provides a comprehensive account of domain-specific instruments or scales that have been developed for, or applied to, studies of cancer patients. The domains for which many 'free-standing' instruments are available include psychological well-being, anxiety, depression, mood, cognitive impairment, adjustment, coping, self-concept, self-esteem, body image, life satisfaction and social support. Bowling cautions against incorporating large numbers of domains into a single instrument or battery of instruments – the potential richness of data collected must be balanced against the burden to patients and researchers. Problems with compliance and completion are known to be proportional to the length and complexity of the instrument used (Sloan et al., 1998). The aims of the study should, therefore, be taken into consideration and only those domains that are directly relevant should be added to the disease-specific or situation-specific core. In many cases core questionnaires and disease-specific modules may be sufficiently comprehensive and may have well-established subscales for the relevant domains, so that they do not require further supplementation.

Individualized measures

In view of the fact that specific contributors to quality of life vary greatly from individual to individual, it has been suggested that quality of life should be measured with individualized rather than standardized instruments. Individualized instruments, such as the Schedule for the Evaluation of Individual Quality of Life (SEIQoL) (McGee et al., 1991), ask patients to list the specific contributors that are important to them and then rate their current status and satisfaction in these areas. This type of measure may be very useful in clinical settings to ensure that patients receive individualized care according to the priorities that they have identified. However, for research purposes, where we are concerned with measuring the quality of life of groups of people, such detail is not normally required and may create difficulties with interpretation of the data because different people in the group will be rating different domains, and the same individual may be rating different domains if measured at two points in time (Cohen, 2003a).

Questionnaire design

Ferrell (1996) suggests that the way we ask questions about quality of life is critical, e.g. the use of projection techniques in some studies has yielded far richer results than straightforward questions about the impact of disease and treatment of quality of life. Such techniques include asking patients what advice they would give to another patient, or asking family members of a patient with cancer how they would advise another family in a similar situation. This approach may be time-consuming and difficult to use in research studies where sample size is relatively large. The same problem arises with more traditional open-ended questions, such as asking patients to generate their own list of quality-of-life concerns.

To simplify data collection and analysis in population studies, researchers tend to use a standard Likert scale format, where patients are asked to rate various items on a verbal scale from very good to very bad. Numerical rating scales (e.g. 0–10) with verbal anchors at each end are also used and recommended for those who need the questionnaire to be read aloud to them (Cohen and Mount, 1992). Other researchers advocate a visual analogue scale, where patients mark a point along a continuum anchored by two extreme and opposite descriptors, and the distance from one end is measured. Scoring by this method is reported to be more labour intensive and some respondents have difficulty understanding the concept (Fayers and Jones, 1983; Selby and Robertson, 1987). Reviews of quality-of-life instruments, including excerpts that illustrate different designs, are provided by Bowling (1995, pp. 34–60) and Cella (1996).

Scoring of quality-of-life instruments

As quality of life is a multidimensional phenomenon, instruments must measure a range of domains, as previously described. Scores for these domains or subscales are often aggregated into a single quality-of-life score, which may be of interest for some research purposes, but which is not particularly meaningful in many circumstances. An aggregate score says nothing about the patient's state in different domains. The reasons for changes in aggregated scores are, therefore, difficult to interpret. In addition, the aggregate score may remain stable, even though there is great improvement in one domain and great deterioration in another. To avoid this problem, it is generally recommended that a profile of scores for the different domains be reported to allow the positive and negative effects of a given treatment to be identified, thereby providing more meaningful and comprehensive information to both the researcher and the clinician, e.g. conservative surgery may lead to a better body image, but increased fear of recurrence. If aggregate ratings are used, these items may cancel each other out, leaving no measurable net gain or loss (Aaronson, 1990).

Asking patients to rate the relative importance or saliency of each item or domain has been put forward as one solution to the problem of accounting for the different contributions that subscales and items make to the aggregate score. This approach is particularly helpful for the clinician, but the trade-off is a more cumbersome scoring system for the researcher and greater burden to the patient, as a result of long and unwieldy instruments. Weightings are used in a number of quality-of-life instruments such as the FACT (Cella et al., 1993), the Ferrans and Powers Quality of Life Index (Ferrans, 1990), the SEIQoL (McGee et al., 1991) and the original version of the Hospice Quality of Life Index (McMillan and Mahon, 1994). The FACT attempts to reduce the instrument burden by measuring the importance of each domain, rather than each item.

The trade-off between richness of data and instrument burden associated with weightings has led to some debate among researchers. It has been suggested that weightings are not worth the trouble when measuring the quality of life of groups of patients, e.g. McMillan and Mahon (1994), using the

Hospice Quality of Life Index, revealed that the correlation between the raw scores and the weighted scores was 0.96, suggesting that weighting does not contribute enough new information to justify the added burden to the patient (although there are problems with the calculation of the weighted scores in this study). However, when quality-of-life measures are used by nurses to identify issues that concern individual patients, important weightings may be invaluable in helping to prioritize goals for care-giving, and for monitoring responses to interventions and changes over the disease trajectory.

Psychometric properties of quality-of-life instruments

The basic criteria that quality-of-life instruments should meet are acceptability, reliability, validity and responsiveness to change. It is beyond the scope of this chapter to elaborate on these standard psychometric parameters and readers are referred to textbooks on research methods for further information (Nunnally and Bernstein, 1994; Streiner and Norman, 1995).

Practical issues in measurement

Two concerns that must be considered when studying quality of life are the burden placed on researchers and on patients. Most researchers and clinicians are sensitive to the potential for patient burden when completing questionnaires. However, clinicians may overestimate the negative impact on the patient, because there are positive aspects of patients' participation that may be unrecognized or undervalued, e.g. patients often express their appreciation for the opportunity to talk about their quality of life (Aaronson, 1990; Cohen et al., 1995; Ferrell, 1996), or to help others like them in the future. Furthermore, the unnecessary exclusion of patients misclassified as too ill to participate can lead to serious bias in sampling and denies such groups the potential benefits that could be gained from inclusion in research studies.

Data collection for research purposes should be funded and planning should be undertaken in close consultation with clinical staff, to ensure that all phases of the research protocol are feasible. For the purposes of research, the quality-of-life data should ideally be collected by a person who is not a member of the patient's treatment team, because the patient's answers may be influenced by a desire to please the staff. When used for clinical purposes, staff burden in collecting data and continued follow-up of patients must be considered. In future, better use of technology may facilitate routine quality-of-life assessment by clinicians, with the aim of improving communication among patients and health professionals. In turn, this may lead to improvements in care, based on a shared understanding of the patients' problems, anticipated needs and strengths, e.g. research on the use of computer touch screens to produce rapid summaries of patients' self-reported symptoms and psychological status before consultation with the oncologist is currently being undertaken at the Peter McCallum Cancer Institute, Melbourne, Australia (Sue-Anne McLachlan, Principal Investigator, personal communication). This approach aims to facilitate communication about patients' problems and needs, enabling the oncologist to address and monitor patients' concerns during each consultation. The use of computer touch screens to measure quality of life in cancer patients is reported to be well accepted by cancer patients and reliable (Buxton et al., 1998; Velikova et al., 1999).

Some problems with measurement

Unfortunately, research on measurement of quality of life has not been adequately linked to research on the theoretical foundations of the phenomenon (Ganz et al., 1988, King et al., 1997). De Boer et al. (1999), in their review of quality of life in head and neck cancer patients, report that, although there are now at least 14 independently developed modules and questionnaires specific to cancer of the head and neck that measure aspects of quality of life, few are in general use and only one study describes the development of a theoretical model for quality of life in patients with this cancer. De Boer et al. (1999) recommend the development of theoretical models and using them to link quality of life, integrated care and coping.

The importance of using valid and reliable quality-of-life measures has been highlighted by Fallowfield (1996) in relation to the emerging trend towards use of such measures as prognostic indicators. If decisions about eligibility for treatments in a cost-conscious health environment are made on the basis of quality-of-life assessments, it is even more important that we have confidence in the validity, reliability and responsiveness of quality-of-life instruments and the theoretical foundations on which they are built. Given the current state of development of these instruments, it would be dangerous to use quality-of-life results as the primary indicator of whether or not a specific intervention should be funded.

The content validity of many instruments is still in question in some situations. All relevant domains must be included; otherwise the instrument lacks validity and interpretation of results is fraught with difficulties, e.g. the assumption that physical status declines as the disease progresses is often reasonable, but the assumption that quality of life is, therefore, lower for people with advanced disease ignores the important contribution of the psychological, social and spiritual domains, which tend to become more important with impending death (Cohen and Mount, 1992; Mount and Cohen, 1995). If these latter domains are not assessed adequately, the interpretation of findings is misleading, because it is based on limited dimensions of a multidimensional construct.

Whom should we ask about patients' quality of life?

This question relates to two distinct aspects of quality-of-life assessment: instrument design and instrument administration. First, when selecting a particular instrument for measuring quality of life we should consider the extent to which the patient's perspective has shaped its development. Gill and Feinstein (1994) have suggested that researchers appear to be far more concerned with 'psychometric elegance' than with the need to incorporate patients' values and preferences into quality-of-life assessments. Many instruments lack simple face validity from patients' perspectives and could be improved by giving patients the opportunity to add their own items to existing scales and to indicate the extent to which items are personally important to them (Gill and Feinstein, 1994). It is possible that instruments with items that are chosen based on analysis of patient interviews have sufficient validity to measure the quality of life of groups of people and also that individual weightings of importance are not necessary. This remains to be tested.

According to Grant et al. (1990) some patient-generated items are included in most quality-of-life tools, although at the time none had been derived solely from qualitative research. Cohen et al. (1997b) have recently developed a revised version of the McGill Quality of Life Questionnaire for palliative care patients, based entirely on qualitative data from interviews conducted in two languages – English and French. Other instruments based on qualitative interviews with cancer patients include the

Quality of Life–Cancer Survivors (Ferrell et al., 1995b), the FACT (Cella et al., 1993), the Quality of Life Index (Padilla et al., 1983) and the revised McGill Quality of Life Questionnaire (Quality of Life in Life-Threatening Illness or QOLLTI – under evaluation by one of the authors – SRC).

Turning now to instrument administration, we need to consider the question of who should provide the information about a patient's quality of life. In other words, to what extent should an instrument rely on self-reported patient ratings (e.g. the EORTC modules), as opposed to being completed by health professionals (e.g. the Spitzer Quality of Life Index – Spitzer et al., 1981)? Given the previous discussion about the subjective and dynamic nature of quality-of-life perceptions, it seems logical to use patient self-reports. However, there may be situations in which other perspectives may be helpful or, indeed, the only alternative. Furthermore, even patient self-reports may sometimes be distorted. Therefore, an awareness of the strengths and limitations of different perspectives may help nurses to interpret quality-of-life assessments with greater sensitivity.

Patient self-reports

It is generally considered that the patient's perspective of quality of life is the most valid and should be used wherever possible (Sprangers and Aaronson, 1992). However, there are a number of factors that may influence patient self-ratings. First, patients may not fully disclose negative feelings in an effort to appear positive or appreciative of the care that they are receiving. This is often referred to as 'social desirability' and its effect can be measured by the concurrent administration of one of a variety of social desirability instruments (Bowling, 1995, p. 294). Second, patients may not disclose the extent of their physical and emotional suffering in order to protect their family members from distress (Lobchuk et al., 1997; Kristjanson et al., 1998). Third, as previously discussed, patient self-reports may reflect changing internal standards against which patients evaluate their own quality of life. Although this gives a true measure of quality of life (a perception of well-being), specific measures of symptom intensity may be required if changes in these are of primary interest. Fourth, patients may misunderstand the purpose of the research study or the clinical interview and deliberately frame their responses either to avoid or to promote anticipated changes to their care (Bernhard et al., 1995).

Another limitation of patient self-reports arises when patients are too frail, ill or confused to convey their feelings and concerns to others. In these situations, the potential value of proxy ratings by healthcare professionals or family members cannot be overlooked, although the limitations of proxy reports, described below, must be taken into account in interpretation of the results.

Healthcare professionals' perceptions

In general, healthcare workers tend to perceive patients' quality of life more negatively than patients (Blazeby et al., 1995, Grassi et al., 1996; Sloan et al., 1998). However, there is not complete agreement, e.g. Bjordal et al. (1995) reported that the treating surgeon consistently overestimated the patients' assessment of their quality of life after treatment for head and neck cancer. Despite such inconsistencies, a review of the use of proxy raters in quality-of-life research has identified a number of clear trends, including: (1) healthcare providers and significant others tend to underestimate patients' quality of life; (2) healthcare providers and significant others are comparable in terms of their accuracy in rating patients' quality of life; and (3) proxy ratings are more accurate when concrete and observable information is sought (Sprangers and Aaronson, 1992).

Inconsistent results obtained from studies of proxy ratings may be partly explained by differences in research design and instruments used to measure quality of life. Instruments that differ in the balance of physical and psychosocial domains may influence the outcomes of agreement studies, e.g. Brunelli et al. (1998) confirmed previous studies showing that agreements among palliative care patients and healthcare providers were higher for physical symptoms than for psychosocial and cognitive symptoms, and that there was a greater agreement on the absence, rather than the presence, of a problem. Blazeby et al. (1995) observed that there was a greater reliance on physical functioning by doctors, compared with psychosocial factors by patients, when rating quality of life. Differences in disease and symptom acuity may also influence congruence ratings. Sloan et al. (1998) found that physicians' assessment of the quality of life for advanced colorectal patients was better at the extreme levels of the scale.

These studies illustrate the importance of seeking more detailed information about factors that may contribute to lack of agreement between patient and proxy ratings. Such detail may help to resolve the inconsistencies observed in either over- or underestimation of patient ratings by proxies in different studies. To date, no specific characteristics of patients or proxies have been identified for which the degree of agreement has improved (Brunelli et al., 1998). However, research in this area is scarce and further studies are warranted, particularly in view of evidence that nurses and oncologists can improve their ability to rate patients' symptoms over time (Larson et al., 1993; Grassi et al., 1996).

Family caregivers' perceptions

Studies on family members' ability to rate patients' quality of life are limited and have yielded conflicting results (Grassi et al., 1996). In the related area of symptom distress ratings, research findings indicate that family caregivers may be reasonable proxies for assessing symptom distress (Lobchuk et al., 1997; Kristjanson et al., 1998). This area of research has highlighted the need to be aware of family dynamics that might confound the interpretation of congruence ratings. Although these factors have been discussed in relation to symptom distress (Lobchuk et al., 1997; Kristjanson et al., 1998), they may apply equally to quality-of-life assessments.

Patients may underreport negative feelings in an effort to protect the family caregiver from knowing about their suffering. Family caregivers may deny or minimize observations because they lack confidence in their ability to deal with the patient's suffering. They may overestimate the patient's distress by projecting their own suffering on to the patient or their ratings may be affected by personal feelings about how much suffering is expected in such situations. Outcomes may be affected by the settings in which the studies are undertaken, e.g. home care settings may be associated with better agreement as a result of close physical contact between patient and caregiver, in which case the length and quality of the relationship and length of the caregiving role may be important factors. Epstein et al. (1989) have shown that the frequency and quality of contact within the family are crucial factors affecting the ability of family members to empathize with the ill relative and to rate the patient's experience of symptoms accurately. Dar et al. (1992) showed that, when patients were relatively stoic (and thus likely to underreport pain), their spouses tended to rate the patients' pain more highly, compared with patients' self-reports.

Nurses have the potential to help family members to assess patients' symptoms and quality of life more accurately and to become more confident and skilled in managing their care. However, research is needed to guide the development of appropriate educational interventions. To this end, studies on the cues used by family caregivers to assess patient symptoms have been undertaken to a limited extent (Lobchuk and Kristjanson, 1997; Kristjanson et al., 1998).

Au et al. (1994) have demonstrated the positive effect of training caregivers to increase their ability to assess patients' pain. Further studies are required to identify characteristics of caregivers and other variables that may enhance or impair assessment, particularly for emotional aspects that are more difficult to assess, and to develop education resources that address the needs of different patient groups.

In summary, although the aim in quality-of-life assessments should be for patient-based self-report questionnaires (with interviewer assistance if required), there is also a need for valid and reliable instruments that can be completed by proxies such as healthcare workers or family members, when patients are too ill or frail to respond. The difficulty in evaluating such instruments lies in the fact that we currently rely on congruence studies conducted with patients who are well enough to participate in research and who are, therefore, able to provide verbal and other cues that may assist others in their assessment. The extent to which caregivers can learn to assess symptom distress and quality of life accurately using more intuitive or subjective cues needs to be evaluated.

When should quality of life be measured?

There are many time points along the cancer trajectory at which patients may experience major changes in the perception of quality of life (Aaronson, 1990; Ferrell, 1996). These stages include diagnosis, treatment, later post-treatment (impact of altered lifestyle), recurrence and terminal illness. Embedded within this broader framework are the day-to-day fluctuations in events, symptoms and moods, from which arise the 'good day/bad day' perceptions (Cohen and Mount, 1996). For this reason, it is important to ask patients how they rate their quality of life over appropriate time spans, e.g. in the acute stages, one could ask about quality of life during the preceding weeks, whereas during specific treatments, or the terminal phase of illness, where patients may experience rapid fluctuations in their condition, a time span of 2–3 days is more appropriate (Cohen and Mount, 1992).

Ferrell (1996) notes that, across all of her studies on psychological well-being in cancer survivors, the survey item rated as causing the most distress was communication of the initial cancer diagnosis. Further along the continuum, there is also evidence from Ferrell's work that quality-of-life concerns in long-term survivors continue far beyond the completion of treatment, despite patients' knowledge of a favourable prognosis. These observations reinforce the importance of longitudinal measurement of quality of life. The interpretation and clinical implications of findings from such longitudinal studies, however, present considerable challenges when one takes into account the inherent dynamism of individual quality-of-life perceptions, and the capacity of patients to adjust their expectations according to changing circumstances.

To date, there is a paucity of longitudinal studies on quality of life (King et al., 1997), although limited follow-up studies have recently been published for patients with head and neck cancer (Gritz et al., 1999) and colorectal cancer (Ulander et al., 1997). In addition, Sprangers et al. (1995) have reviewed 17 studies on aspects of quality of life predominantly concerned with sexual function of patients after surgery for colorectal cancer. Some researchers have drawn attention to the need for prospective studies of healthy people to establish a disease-free baseline and to identify aspects of quality of life that may be unique to the cancer experience (King et al., 1997; Ulander et al., 1997).

Future directions

There appears to be agreement among a number of researchers that we must work towards the refinement of a conceptual model for quality of life to provide a solid theoretical foundation for its assessment (King et al., 1997). This model must be grounded in data collected from the patients themselves about which domains are important to their quality of life. Researchers should be cautioned against the unlimited development of new instruments when many are already available that could benefit from refinement rather than duplication. Similarly, the demand for quality-of-life instruments suitable for clinical settings may often be satisfied by modification of existing research instruments, rather than the creation of new ones (King et al., 1997). For the purposes of clinical use rather than research, we need to determine whether standardized instruments are sufficiently valid, reliable and sensitive to change, or whether individualized instruments, for which the patient nominates his or her own domains, are required. Similarly, we need further studies to determine whether the individualized measures are useful for studying the quality of life of groups of people

Attention to cultural influences on quality-of-life measurement is urgently needed, to reflect the wide variations in philosophies of life, health, illness, death and family among different cultures (Ferrell, 1996). This goes beyond translating existing instruments into different languages. Although valuable information may be gained by this approach, the interpretations of differences and similarities are limited by the cultural perspective within which the research instrument has been designed. There is a need to consider how cultural differences may influence the conceptual domains through which we define quality of life and the priorities given to different domains by different cultures across the disease trajectory. Therefore, qualitative and descriptive quantitative approaches that capture individual perspectives are warranted. A preliminary study by Chaturvedi (1991) on what is important to quality of life in Indians is an important step forward.

Cultural sensitivity also extends to the issues surrounding gender differences and similarities, according to Dibble et al. (1998). These researchers have questioned the current consensus that quality of life encompasses the same dimensions for both sexes. Their empirically derived dimensions of quality of life differed for men and women; the two dimensions for women were psychosocial well-being and physical competence (physical attributes and abilities), whereas the two dimensions for men were vitality and personal resources. Further research is necessary to confirm these findings and to determine the impact of this conceptual shift on the design and analysis of quality-of-life studies.

Improved methods are needed for assessing quality of life when patients are too ill or frail to respond. As previously discussed, there is encouraging evidence that health professionals and family caregivers can improve the accuracy of their assessments of patients' quality of life. However, to date, most research on the use of proxy ratings has focused on measuring the extent of agreement between raters and patients, rather than studying the characteristics of patients and proxies and the underlying processes that influence the accuracy of ratings. Such information is required to guide the development of appropriate educational interventions.

Quality of life in children with cancer is an area that needs continued attention, particularly as new treatments offering prolonged survival are developed. In the last decade, researchers have worked on the development of definitions and instruments for quality-of-life assessment in children and adolescents with cancer (Hinds, 1990; Rosenbaum et al., 1990; Bradlyn et al., 1993).

Finally, there is a need for research on how nursing care may impact on various dimensions of quality of life, so that nurses can work collaboratively with their patients and other health-care professionals to provide optimum care.

Conclusion

Although there is still considerable debate about conceptual definitions and measurement issues relating to quality of life, there is general agreement about the importance of measuring quality of life as an outcome at all stages of the cancer experience. With the continuing evolution of knowledge about the theoretical foundations of quality of life comes the need to integrate new findings into nursing education, practice and research. Nurses have already made significant contributions to quality-of-life research (Ferrans, 1990; Hinds, 1990; Padilla, 1993; Ferrell, 1996; King et al., 1997). In their unique role as health professionals with the most intimate and prolonged contact with patients and their families, they are ideally placed to take a leading role in expanding our knowledge of quality-of-life theory and applying this theory to practice.

Acknowledgements

The authors gratefully acknowledge the literature search assistance of Aurora Popescu, financial support from Edith Cowan University and salary support for SRC from the Medical Research Council of Canada.

References

Aaronson NK (1990) Quality of life research in cancer clinical trials: a need for common rules and language. Oncology 4: 59–66.

Aaronson NK, Ahmedzai S, Bergman B (1993) The EORTC QLQ-C30: A quality of life instrument for use in international clinical trials in oncology. Journal of the National Cancer Institute 85: 365–376.

Allison PJ, Locker D, Feine JS (1997) Quality of life: a dynamic construct. Social Science and Medicine 45: 221–230.

Au E, Loprinzi CL, Dhodpakar M et al. (1994) Regular use of a verbal pain scale improves the understanding of oncology inpatient pain intensity. Journal of Clinical Oncology 12: 2751–2755.

Bandura A (1982) Self-efficacy mechanism in human agency. American Psychologist 37: 47.

Belcher AE, Dettmore D, Holzemer SP (1989) Spirituality and sense of well-being in persons with AIDS. Holistic Nurse Practitioner 3: 16–25.

Bernhard J, Gusset H, Hurny C (1995) Quality of life assessment in cancer clinical trials: an intervention by itself? Supportive Care in Cancer 3: 66–71.

Bjordal K, Freng A, Thorvik J, Kaasa S (1995) Patient self-reported and clinician-rated quality of life in head and neck cancer patients: a cross-sectional study. Oral Oncology, European Journal of Cancer 31B: 235–241.

Bjordal K, Hammerlid E, Ahlner-Elmqvist M et al. (1999) Quality of life in head and neck cancer patients: validation of the European Organization for Research and Treatment of Cancer Quality of Life Questionnaire–H&N35. Journal of Clinical Oncology 17: 1008–1019.

Blazeby JM, Williams MH, Brookes ST, Alderson D, Farndon JR (1995) Quality of life measurement in patients with oesophageal cancer. Gut 37: 505–508.

Blijham GH, Labianca R, Bleiberg H (1997) Should patients with advanced colorectal cancer be treated with chemotherapy. European Journal of Cancer 33: 815–824.

Bowling A (1995) Measuring Disease: A Review of Disease-Specific Quality of Life Measurement Scales. Buckingham: Open University Press.

Bradburn NM (1969) The Structure of Psychological Well-Being. Chicago: Aldine Publishing Co.

Bradlyn AS, Harris CV, Warner JE, Ritchey AK, Zaboy K (1993) An investigation of the validity of the quality of well-being scale with pediatric oncology patients. Health Psychology 12: 246–250.

Brady MJ, Peterman AH, Fitchett G, Mo M, Cella D (1999) A case for including spirituality in quality of life measurement in oncology. Psycho-oncology 8: 417–428.

Breetvelt IS, Van Dam FSAM (1991) Underreporting by cancer patients: the case of response-shift. Social Science in Medicine 32: 981–987.

Bremnes RM, Adersen K, Wist EA (1995) Cancer patients, doctors and nurses vary in their willingness to undertake cancer chemotherapy. European Journal of Cancer 31A: 1955–1959.

Brunelli C, Costantini M, Di Giulio P et al. (1998) Quality-of-life evaluation: When do terminal cancer patients and health-care providers agree. Journal of Pain and Symptom Management 15: 151–158.

Buxton J, White M, Osaba D (1998) Patients' experiences using a computerized program with a touch-sensitive video monitor for the assessment of health-related quality of life. Quality of Life Research 7: 513–519.

Byock IR, Merriman MP (1998) Measuring quality of life for patients with terminal illness: the Missoula - VITAS Quality of Life Index. Palliative Medicine 12:2 31-244.

Calman KC (1984) Quality of life in cancer patients: an hypothesis. Journal of Medical Ethics 10: 124-127.

Campbell A, Converse PE, Rodgers WL (1976) The quality of American life. New York: Russell Sage Foundation.

Cantril H (1965) The pattern of human concerns. New Jersey: Rutgers University Press.

Carver CS, Scheier MF (1982) Control theory: a useful conceptual framework for personality - social, clinical and health psychology. Psychological Bulletin 91(1): 111-135.

Cassileth BR, Lusk EJ, Tenaglia ANA (1982) Psychological comparison of patients with malignant melanomas and other dermatological diseases. American Academy of Dermatology 7: 742-746.

Cella DF (1994) Quality of life: Concepts and definition. Journal of Pain and Symptom Management 9: 186-192.

Cella DF (1995) Measuring quality of life in palliative care. Seminars in Oncology 22: 73-81.

Cella DF (1996) Quality of life outcomes: measurement and validation. Oncology (Huntington) 1: 233-246.

Cella DF, Tulsky DS, Gray G et al. (1993) The Functional Assessment of Cancer Therapy (FACT) Scale: development and validation of the general measure. Journal of Clinical Oncology 11: 570-579.

Chaturvedi SK (1991) What's important for quality of life to Indians - in relation to cancer. Social Science in Medicine 33: 91-94.

Cohen SR (2003a) Assessing quality of life in palliative care. In: Bruera E, Portnoy R (eds), Research in Palliative Care: Methodologies and outcomes. Oxford: Oxford University Press: 231-241.

Cohen SR (2003b) Quality of life as an outcome measure in palliative care. In: Bruera E, Portnoy R (eds), Topics in Palliative Care, Vol 5. Oxford: Oxford University Press: 137-156.

Cohen SR, Mount BM (1992) Quality of life in terminal illness: Defining and measuring subjective well-being in the dying. Journal of Palliative Care 8: 40-45.

Cohen SR, Mount BM (1996) Good days, bad days: Quantitative and qualitative differences for oncology patients. Journal of Palliative Care 12: 62.

Cohen SR, Mount BM, Strobel MG, Bui F (1995) The McGill Quality of Life Questionnaire: a measure of quality of life appropriate for people with advanced disease. A preliminary study of validity and acceptability. Palliative Medicine 9: 207-219.

Cohen SR, Mount BM, Tomas J, Mount L (1996) Existential well-being is an important determinant of quality of life: evidence from the McGill Quality of Life Questionnaire. Cancer 77: 576-586.

Cohen SR, Bultz BD, Clarke J et al. (1997a) Well-being at the end of life: Part 1. A research agenda for psychosocial and spiritual aspects of care from the patient's perspective. Cancer Prevention and Control 1: 334-342.

Cohen SR, Mount BM, Bruera E, Provost M, Rowe J, Tong K (1997b) Validity of the McGill Quality of Life Questionnaire in the palliative care setting: a multi-centre Canadian study demonstrating the importance of the existential domain. Palliative Medicine 11: 3-20.

Costa PT, McCrae RR (1980) Influence of extraversion and neuroticism on subjective well-being: happy and unhappy people. Journal of Personality and Social Psychology 38: 668–678.

Coward DD (1994) Meaning and purpose in the lives of persons with AIDS. Public Health Nurse, 331–336.

Dar R, Beach CM, Barden PL, Cleeland CS (1992) Cancer pain in the marital system: A study of patients and their spouses. Journal of Pain and Symptom Management 7: 87–93.

De Boer MF, McCormick LK, Pruyn JFA, Ryckman RM, van den Borne BW (1999) Physical and psychosocial correlates of head and neck cancer: A review of the literature. Otolaryngology – Head and Neck Surgery 120: 427–436.

de Haes JCJM, van Knippenberg FCE (1985) The quality of life of cancer patients: a review of the literature. Social Science in Medicine 20: 809–817.

Decker SD, Schultz R (1985) Correlates of life satisfaction and depression in middle-aged and elderly spinal cord injured patients. American Journal of Occupational Therapy 39: 740–745.

Dibble SL, Padilla GV, Dodd MJ, Miaskowski C (1998) Gender differences in the dimensions of quality of life. Oncology Nursing Forum 25: 577–583.

Donovan K, Sanson-Fisher RW, Redman S (1989) Measuring quality of life in cancer patients. Journal of Clinical Oncology 7: 959–968.

Eischens MJ, Elliott BA, Elliott TE (1998) Two hospice quality of life surveys: a comparison. American Journal of Hospice and Palliative Care 15: 143–148.

Epstein AM, Hall JA, Togneti J, Son LH, Conant L (1989) Using proxies to evaluate quality of life. Medical Care 27: S91–98.

Evans RW (1991) Quality of life. The Lancet 338: 636.

Fallowfield L (1996) Quality of quality-of-life data. The Lancet 348: 421–422.

Fayers PM, Jones DR (1983) Measuring and analysing quality of life in cancer clinical trials: A review. Statistics in Medicine 2: 429–446.

Ferrans CE (1990) Development of a quality of life index for patients with cancer. Oncology Nursing Forum 17: 15–21.

Ferrans CE, Powers MJ (1985) Quality of Life Index: development and psychometric properties. Advances in Nursing Science 8: 15–24.

Ferrell BR (1996) The quality of lives: 1,525 voices of cancer. Oncology Nursing Forum 23: 909–916.

Ferrell B, Wisdom C, Wenzl C (1989) QOL as an outcome variable in the management of cancer pain. Cancer 63: 2321–2327.

Ferrell B, Grant M, Schmidt G et al. (1992a) The meaning of quality of life for bone marrow transplant survivors. Part 1: The impact of bone marrow transplant on quality of life. Cancer Nursing 15: 153–160.

Ferrell B, Grant M, Schmidt G, Rhiner M, Whitehead C, Fonbuena P, Forman S (1992b) The meaning of quality of life for bone marrow transplant survivors. Part 1: The impact of bone marrow transplant on QOL. Cancer Nursing 15: 247–253.

Ferrell B, Dow KH, Leigh S (1995a) QOL in cancer survivors. Oncology Nursing Forum 21: 377.

Ferrell BR, Dow KH, Leigh S, Ly J, Gulasekaram P (1995b) Quality of life in long-term cancer survivors. Oncology Nursing Forum 22: 915–926.

Festinger L (1954) A theory of social comparison processes. Human Relations 7: 117–140.

Foltz AT (1987) The influence of cancer on self-concept and life quality. Seminars in Oncology Nursing 3: 303–312.

Fryback PB (1993) Health for people with a terminal diagnosis. Nursing Science Quarterly 6: 147–159.

Ganz PA, Haskell CM, Figlin RA, La Soto N, Siau J (1988) Estimating the quality of life in a clinical trial of patients with metastatic lung cancer using the Karnofsky Performance Status and the Functional Living Index – Cancer. Cancer 61: 849–856.

Gill TM, Feinstein AR (1994) A critical appraisal of the quality of quality-of-life measurements. Journal of the American Medical Association 272: 619–626.

Golembiewski RT, Billingsley K, Yeager S (1976) Measuring change and persistence in human affairs: types of change generated by OD designs. Journal of Applied Behavioural Science 12: 133–157.

Gotay CC (1985) Why me? Attributions and adjustments by cancer patients and their mates at two stages in the disease process. Social Science and Medicine 20: 825–831.

Gough IR, Furnival CM, Schilder I, Grove W (1983) Assessment of the quality of life of patients with advanced cancer. European Journal of Cancer and Clinical Oncology 19: 1161–1165.

Grant MM, Padilla GV, Ferrell BR, Rhiner M (1990) Assessment of quality of life with a single instrument. Seminars in Oncology Nursing 6: 260–270.

Grant M, Ferrell B, Schmidt GM, Fonbuena P, Niland JC, Forman SJ (1992) Measurement of quality of life in bone marrow transplantation survivors. Quality of Life Research 1: 375–384.

Grassi L, Indelli M, Maltoni M, Falcini F, Fabbri L, Indelli R (1996) Quality of life of homebound patients with advanced cancer: Assessments by patients, family members, and oncologists. Journal of Psychosocial Oncology 14: 31–45.

Gritz ER, Carmack CL, de Moor C et al. (1999) First year after head and neck cancer: Quality of life. Journal of Clinical Oncology 17: 352–360.

Helson H (1964) Adaptation Level Theory. New York: Harper & Row.

Heyink J (1993) Adaptation and well-being. Psychological Reports 73: 1331–1342.

Highfield M (1992) Spiritual health of oncology patients: Nurse and patient perspectives. Cancer Nursing 15: 1–8.

Hinds PS (1990) Quality of life in children and adolescents with cancer. Seminars in Oncology Nursing 6: 285–291.

Hyland ME (1992) A reformulation of quality of life for medical science. Quality of Life Research 1: 267–272.

Hyland ME, Kenyon CAP, Jacobs PA (1994) Sensitivity of quality of life domains and constructs to longitudinal change in a clinical trial comparing salmeterol with placebo in asthmatics. Quality of Life Research 3: 121–126.

Kagawa-Singer M (1993) Redefining health: living with cancer. Social Science and Medicine 37: 295–304.

Kahn D, Steeves R (1993) Spiritual well-being: A review of the research literature. Quality of Life: A Nursing Challenge 2: 260–264.

King CR, Haberman M, Berry DL et al. (1997) Quality of life and the cancer experience: The state-of-the-knowledge. Oncology Nursing Forum 24: 27–41.

Kreitler S, Chaitchick S, Rapoport Y, Kreitler H, Algor R (1993) Life satisfaction and health in cancer patients, orthopedic patients and healthy individuals. Social Science and Medicine 36: 547–556.

Kristjanson L, Nikoletti S, Porock D, Smith M, Lobchuk M, Pedler P (1998) Congruence between patients' and family caregivers' perceptions of symptom distress in patients with terminal cancer. Journal of Palliative Care 14: 24–32.

Larson PJ, Viele CS, Coleman S, Dibble, SL, Cebulski C (1993) Comparison of perceived symptoms of patients undergoing bone marrow transplant and the nurses caring for them. Oncology Nursing Forum 20: 81–88.

Lazarus RS, Folkman S (1984) Stress, Appraisal and Coping. New York: Springer.

Linder-Petz S (1982) Social psychological determinates of patient satisfaction: A test of five hypotheses. Social Science in Medicine 16: 583–589.

List MA, D'Antonio LL, Cella DF et al. (1996) The Performance Status Scale for Head and Neck Cancer Patients and the Functional Assessment of Cancer Therapy-Head and Neck Scale. A study of utility and validity. Cancer 77: 2294–2301.

Lobchuk M, Kristjanson L (1997) Perceptions of symptom distress in lung cancer patients: II. Behavioral assessment by primary family caregivers. Journal of Pain and Symptom Management 14: 147–156.

Lobchuk MM, Kristjanson L, Degner L, Blood P, Sloan J A (1997) Perceptions of symptom distress in lung cancer patients: I. Congruence between patients and primary family caregivers. Journal of Pain and Symptom Management 14: 136–146.

McGee HM, O'Boyle CA, Hickey A, O'Malley K, Joyce CRB (1991) Assessing the quality of life of the individual: the SEIQoL with a healthy and a gastroenterology unit population. Psychological Medicine 21: 749–759.

McMillan SC, Mahon M (1994) Measuring quality of life in hospice patients using a newly developed Hospice Quality of Life Index. Quality of Life Research 3: 437–447.

Maslow AH (1954) Motivation and Personality. New York: Harper & Row.

Mechanic D (1962) The concept of illness behaviour. Journal of Chronic Diseases 17: 189–194.

Mishel MH (1988) Uncertainty in illness. Journal of Nursing Scholarship 20: 225–232.

Mount BM, Cohen SR (1995) Quality of life in the face of life-threatening illness: What should we be measuring? Current Oncology 2: 121–125.

Najman JM, Levine S (1981) Evaluating the impact of medical care and technologies on the quality of life: a review and critique. Social Science and Medicine 15: 107–115.

Neuman B (1974) The Betty Neuman health care systems model: a total person approach to patient problems. In: Riehl JP, Roy C (eds), Conceptual Models for Nursing Practice. New York: Appleton-Century-Crofts, pp. 94–104.

Nunnally JC, Bernstein IH (1994). Psychometric Theory, 3rd edn. New York: McGraw-Hill.

O'Connor A, Wicker C, Germino B (1990) Understanding the cancer patient's search for meaning. Cancer Nursing 3: 167–175.

Padilla GV (1993) State of the art in quality of life research. Communicating Nursing Research 26: 71–80.

Padilla GV, Grant MM (1985) Quality of life as a cancer nursing outcome variable. Advances in Nursing Science 8: 45–60.

Padilla GV, Presant C, Grant MM, Metter G, Lipsett J, Heide F (1983) Quality of life index for patients with cancer. Research in Nursing and Health 6: 117–126.

Padilla GV, Ferrell B, Grant MM, Rhiner M (1990) Defining the content domain of quality of life for cancer patients with pain. Cancer Nursing 13: 108–115.

Padilla GV, Mishel MH, Grant MM (1992) Uncertainty, appraisal and quality of life. Quality of Life Research 1: 155–165.

Pratheepawanit N, Salek MS, Finaly IG (1999) The applicability of quality-of-life assessment in palliative care: comparing two quality-of-life measures. Palliative Medicine 13: 325-334.

Redmond K (1998a) Assessing patients' needs and preferences in the management of advanced colorectal cancer. British Journal of Cancer 77: 5-7.

Redmond K (1998b) Treatment choices in advanced cancer: issues and perspectives. European Journal of Cancer Care 7: 31-39.

Rosenbaum P, Cadman D, Kerpalani H (1990) Pediatrics: Assessing quality of life. In: Spilker B (ed.), Quality of Life Assessments in Clinical Trials. New York: Raven Press, pp. 205-215.

Roy DJ (1992) Measurement in the service of compassion. Journal of Palliative Care 8: 3-4.

Scheier MF, Carver CS (1985) Optimism, coping and health: assessment and implications of generalised outcome expectancies. Health Psychology 4: 219-247.

Scheier MF, Carver CS (1987) Dispositional optimism and recovery from coronary artery bypass surgery: the beneficial effects upon physical and psychological well-being. Journal of Personality 55: 169-210.

Schipper H, Clinch J, McMurray A, Levitt M (1984) Measuring the quality of life of cancer patients: the Functional Living Index – Cancer: development and validation. Journal of Clinical Oncology 2: 472-483.

Selby P, Robertson B (1987) Measurement of quality of life in patients with cancer. Cancer Surveys 6: 521-542.

Sloan JA, Loprinzi CL, Kuross SA et al. (1998) Randomized comparison of four tools measuring overall quality of life in patients with advanced cancer. Journal of Clinical Oncology 16: 3662-3673.

Spitzer WO, Dobson AJ, Hall J et al. (1981) Measuring quality of life of cancer patients: A concise QL-index for use by physicians. Journal of Chronic Diseases 34: 585-597.

Sprangers MAG (1996) Response-shift bias: a challenge to the assessment of patients' quality of life in cancer clinical trials. Cancer Treatment Reviews 22: 55-62.

Sprangers MAG, Aaronson NK (1992) The role of health care providers and significant others in evaluating the quality of life of patients with chronic disease: A review. Journal of Clinical Epidemiology 45: 743-760.

Sprangers M, Taal BG, Aaronson N, te Velde A (1995) Quality of life in colorectal cancer – stoma vs. nonstoma patients. Diseases of the Colon and Rectum 38: 361-369.

Sprangers MAG, Cull A, Groenvold M, Bjordal K, Blazeby J, Aaronson NK (1998) The European Organization for Research and Treatment of Cancer approach to developing questionnaire modules: an update and overview. Quality of Life Research 7: 291-300.

Sprangers MA, te Velde A, Aaronson NK (1999) The construction and testing of the EORTC colorectal cancer-specific quality of life questionnaire module (QLQ-CR38). European Organization for Research and Treatment of Cancer Study Group on Quality of Life. European Journal of Cancer 35: 238-247.

Sterkenburg CA (1996) A reliability and validity study of the McMaster Quality of Life Scale (MQLS) for a palliative population. Journal of Palliative Care 12: 18-25.

Streiner DL, Norman GR (1995) Health Measurement Scales: A practical guide to their development and use. New York: Oxford University Press.

Ulander K, Jeppsson B, Grahn G (1997) Quality of life and independence in activities of daily living preoperatively and at follow-ups in patients with colorectal cancer. Support Care Cancer 5: 402–409.

Velikova G, Wright EP, Smith AB et al. (1999) Automated collection of quality-of-life data: a comparison of paper and computer touch-screen questionnaires. Journal of Clinical Oncology 17: 998–1007.

Ward WL, Hahn EA, Mo F, Hernandes L, Tulsky DS, Cella D (1999) Reliability and validity of the Functional Assessment of Cancer Therapy - Colorectal (FACT-C) quality of life instrument. Quality of Life Research 8: 181–195.

Watson D, Pennebaker JW (1989) Health complaints, stress, and distress: exploring the central role of negative affectivity. Psychological Reviews 96: 234–254.

Weisman A, Worden AD (1976) The existential plight in cancer: Significance of the first 100 days. International Journal of Psychiatry in Medicine 7: 1–15.

World Health Organization (1998) The World Health Organization Quality of Life Assessment (WHOQOL): development and general psychometric properties. Social Science, Medicine 46: 1569–1585.

Yellen SB, Cella DF, Webster K, Blendowski C, Kaplan E (1997) Measuring fatigue and other anemia-related symptoms with the Functional Assessment of Cancer Therapy (FACT) measurement system. Journal of Pain and Symptom Management 13: 63–74.

CHAPTER 2

Impact of cancer on self-concept

LIZ ASHTON

Having cancer is very stressful – almost as stressful as the death of a close family member and marginally less stressful than marriage (Holmes, 1978). It makes people question their mortality and rethink every area of their life. Normal everyday people become patients. This chapter aims to explore these issues, give some pointers on how to help people on their journey with illness and how to keep enjoying your work as a nurse.

Most people are simply getting on with their lives: work, money, house, care, holidays, pensions, normal worries, traffic jams, scum in the bath, washing-up. People don't want to be ill; it is not convenient. They may have ignored symptoms for some time before the first consultation. Taking the first step towards actually having cancer, rather than being a person with a symptom, is very powerful. People experience a lot of anxiety and understandable concern. They hope to be told there is nothing to worry about, and there may actually be nothing to worry about. When people are reassured by their family doctor, they experience relief. However, some will be referred on to hospital for tests and examinations. Already such people will have begun to examine their sense of self to take on board new information: 'I may have cancer.' 'It is possible that it could happen to me.' They begin to pay more attention to items in magazines and papers, and programmes on TV, beginning a search for information, looking for their symptoms and explanations.

This process is continued and extended throughout patients' early 'cancer career' until they arrive at 'I have cancer', which increases people's vulnerability and affects their self-esteem. People worry about themselves and their family, and will often be depressed and anxious. Cancer can transform people's lives for good or bad. They can start to concentrate on relationships, quality of life and spirituality. They can give and ask for forgiveness, resolving old grudges. People can learn to savour life and live it with a new vigour.

The next portion of this chapter is split into three: assumptions, worries and benefits, taking each in turn and thinking about the impact of cancer on people.

Assumptions

People have various assumptions about themselves. They assume that they will be independent physically and financially, and that they will stay in good health and die as an old person. People hope to see their children grow up, to continue as a sexual being, to be in charge of their lives. Perhaps a lot of this is illusory in any case. People harbour dreams and idle fantasies of glory or wealth, which may not have been articulated but are none the less hard to give up. Having a serious illness challenges all of this. It is not surprising therefore that people find it hard to adjust. Feelings of anger, powerlessness and even rage are expected. Depression and anxiety are common; fleeting feelings of hopelessness and even suicidal ideas can occur. For the majority these feelings will come and go and may be all mixed together, although they can be very powerful. People can adjust quickly even to major changes and some may take on board the new information 'I have cancer' rapidly and without seeming to break their stride. It is the people who fail to adjust and get stuck who can be the most challenging. They are angry and this anger can spill out into other areas of life, such as relationships and even consultations. In consultations, if people are angry the most helpful thing is not to match their anger with your own, but to stay calm: ask people to explain their anger and answer the points if possible; write things down so that people can take the information away.

Assumptions about other people will change as well. People have fixed ways of relating to family and friends. These patterns change; initially, perhaps out of concern, friends and family treat a person with cancer as a patient, or as someone vulnerable and in need of protection. These changes in relationships may not be welcome and can create tension between a person with cancer and the people close to them, e.g. a man with cancer is 'mothered' by his wife, which automatically changes the dynamic of that relationship. The man is no longer a man with a wife as an equal, but a child to be cared for. It must be very hard to lose your role as an autonomous being, even if out of concern. This can be tricky to untangle. People try to behave kindly towards their partners and hope to be helpful. If their efforts are met with anger or resentment then both sides are unhappy. Gently trying to point out to both what is happening can be very helpful. This can be done with the understanding that, when people feel that their lives are under threat, they look for as much consistency as possible. However, it is also important to acknowledge the love, care and concern that is felt for the person with cancer and not to reject that love. Perhaps simply pointing out that the relationship has lost its balance, and the two sides need to find a new equilibrium, is sufficient.

Worries

Having a cancer gives people a whole new repertoire of worries – everyday worries will no longer suffice. People move up to the worry super-league – they have concerns for themselves and others.

For themselves, people want answers to difficult questions:

- How long have I got?
- Will I be in pain?
- What will my scar be like?
- Will I be incontinent?
- Will my bowel habit change?
- Will I need a 'bag'?
- Will I still be able to have sex?
- Will I feel like having sex?
- Will I be in hospital a lot?
- What will happen to my work?

Each of these issues can be like a major or 'trunk' worry, from which flow numerous connected 'branch' worries. People can be left feeling as if their head is spinning. They try to make some sense of the information given to them and go through unending cycles of thoughts which have no answers. If possible, it is good to give simple information clearly, which can be written down and explained. A willingness to go over the same information is helpful because little is taken in at any one time. Of course people have the right to know everything about their illness and information should not be hidden. When answers are not known, e.g. about sexual function after certain procedures, be honest: 'I do not know in your case.' Perhaps you could then go on to explain what happens in similar cases and emphasize that an erection is only part of sexual intimacy. Closeness, affection and warmth are often more important to partners.

The patients will also have worries for and about others:

- What will happen to my wife/husband when I go?
- How will the kids manage without a mum/dad?
- What will my family do for money while I'm off work/when I die?
- How will they cope seeing me frail/becoming unwell?

Sorting out financial affairs such as life assurance policies and pensions is often the most straightforward to organize. The papers can be found, dealt with, put in an envelope, labelled and put somewhere easy to find. The rest will be worried and talked about endlessly. Saying 'I love you' does not become easy as soon as you have cancer, but practice does make it easier. Suggesting to people that they say 'I love you' to their family can spur them on.

> 'I'm sorry I won't be here to see you grow up, I love you.'
> 'I am sorry you will be a widow, I love you.'

This may cause conflict. Perhaps the person with cancer has accepted that he or she is dying when a family is still hoping for a cure. Be honest, explain gently and encourage people to share their good memories with each other.

Benefits

Some people have the amazing ability to transcend difficult and challenging times. They come across as people with peace, grace and humour. They have fully accepted their lot and have moved on, getting on with their life. These people are rare. Most people struggle to come to terms with cancer. In spite of this, there can be benefits to having cancer. It can somehow lift people out of the everyday. People can rediscover their relationships, concentrate on the important things such as enjoyment, pleasure, friendships, take time and be truly alive, more spiritually aware and living for the now. It can allow people to resolve old grudges and forgive themselves. Many people carry burdens that it is never the right time to resolve. Cancer can be that opportunity. You can encourage people in that task simply by being aware of these issues. Ask people to make two lists on the same bit of paper: 'the bad things about having cancer' and 'the good things about having cancer'. If there are no 'good things' then ask what good could come from cancer. What can people do to improve their own lives and the lives of those who love them? If they still look blank, suggest that they ask their family and friends for ideas to make themselves and others happier.

Some people take control in their cancer journey. They read voraciously, search the net, start taking dietary supplements, do visualizations, join groups and become very knowledgeable. They may come across a branch of medicine called psycho-neuroimmunology. This explores mind–body links and sets out to enquire about how the mind can influence the body, particularly through the immune system, e.g. great fear before surgery can be associated with slower and more complicated postoperative recovery (Kiecolt-Glaser et al., 1998). There is evidence that psychological factors can alter the progression of cancer (Garssen and Goodkin, 1999). Feeling that you are in control of your illness seems to amplify the effect of any physical treatments for improving survival (Levy, 1997). Group support can be very good at helping people to feel more in control (Cain et al., 1986).

It would be great if all people's experiences of cancer and support services were positive and life transforming, enabling them to be more in charge of their lives, more alive and more potent members of society.

The next portion of the chapter covers some of the most common psychological problems that occur in people with cancer. There is a brief 'how to' section on communication and perhaps the most important item of all, how to stay healthy while working in a demanding environment.

Common psychological problems

Adjustment reactions, anxiety and depression are the most common psychological disorders. Virtually everyone faced with a diagnosis of cancer will have an emotional response. Up to half would have a formal psychiatric diagnosis if it were appropriate to give people those labels (Derogatis et al., 1983). Short descriptions of adjustment disorder, anxiety and depression (World Health Organization, 1994) follow, with suggestions of what to do or how to get help for these people.

Adjustment disorders

These are simply periods of distress and emotional upset in response to a life event. The distress interferes with everyday life and appears shortly after being stressed. The usual symptoms are mild depression and anxiety, and last for a matter of weeks. People may feel unable to cope and find it difficult to do their everyday planning. These symptoms tend to be self-limiting. The ability to discuss worries with people can be very helpful and reassuring.

Anxiety disorders

There is a whole assortment of anxiety disorders but typically people feel tense and nervous. They may have autonomic symptoms such as palpitations, sweating or a dry mouth. They may experience difficulty breathing, feel they are choking, have churning in the stomach and find it hard to relax. In addition to this general anxiety, people may have panic attacks. A panic attack is a severe episode of anxiety that is unpredictable and occurs spontaneously. People find that these attacks come on suddenly, rapidly reaching a climax. During an attack, people often have a compelling idea that they may be about to die or lose control, or that something terrible is happening to them.

Helping people with anxiety should begin with reassurance and an explanation of the experience. Teaching progressive relaxation and deep breathing exercises is helpful. The first technique involves learning how to relax your body using the breath. First, find a comfortable position or lie down, and then close the eyes. On an in breath, tense the muscles in the feet and, on the out breath, relax them completely; progress up the body, relaxing calves, thighs, abdomen, hands, arms, shoulders, chest and face. Then tense every muscle in the body on an in breath and completely relax on the out breath. Stay relaxed for a few moments before slowly taking a few deeper breaths, after which get up gently. This technique enables people to become more relaxed. It can be done with a person by talking them through the process; it can also be done with groups. Once people have understood the idea, they should practise regularly at home.

Deep breathing is really helpful during panic attacks, because in an attack the breath often becomes shallow and quick. Suggest to patients that they bring their attention to the breath, and instead of a shallow breath take an enormous breath in through the nose and push out the stomach, trying to keep the shoulders level. Slowly breathe out and repeat a few times. It is almost impossible to panic and the technique can be demonstrated very easily.

Most people will manage their anxiety symptoms with such techniques. Sometimes use of antidepressants can be helpful. The SSRIs (selective serotonin reuptake inhibitors) can be used although they are not sedating. If anxiety symptoms are prominent and people are not sleeping, use of an older style tricyclic antidepressant may be appropriate, e.g. amitriptyline. Obviously, general practitioners have a role in helping to find the most useful medications, but patients may appreciate the input of hospital physicians – the surgeon, the physician most directly involved or a psychiatrist.

Depressive disorders

Depressive illness shows itself by a lowering of mood, a reduction in energy and a decrease in activity. People feel very tired all the time and find themselves with less confidence and self-esteem. They may find that they cry a lot. Often sleep patterns and appetite are disturbed. People may feel hopeless and worthless and think that they would be better off dead. Suicide is not common but people contemplating such a course often do not say so. Asking a simple question such as 'what keeps you going?' can be a way to start a conversation about this subject. Another question could be 'what is life worth for you at the moment?'. Even people with very strong suicidal ideas have no intention of killing themselves and have very good reasons to live. If you think a person is depressed, talk to him or her and offer your support. It is also worth considering what else could be appropriate. People may wish for no more than your support or to seek further help. This could be from their GP, medication or group support. It may even be sensible to discuss their troubles with a psychiatrist. To a large extent it depends on what is available in your area. In any case discussion with your colleagues can offer you important support and there are various rating scales that try to look at anxiety and depression. Some, such as the Hospital Anxiety and Depression Scale (HAD) (Zigmond and

Snaith, 1983), can be useful to give some idea of who is really struggling. It was designed for use in non-psychiatric hospital departments. This is a self-report scale, being short at only four items, and people can just tick boxes. It is sensitive to change which has been reasonably researched. It also offers a cut-off point between 'not too bad' and 'really rather unwell'. This can be useful if you are not used to thinking about people's depressive experiences.

There are other, more uncommon psychiatric problems that you may discover when caring for people with cancer. These include such things as confusional states and dissociative disorders. Confusional states or delirium can complicate any physical illness. They present as impaired consciousness, muddled thinking, a disturbed sleep–wake cycle and often vivid visual hallucinations. The causes are many but include electrolyte disturbance, opiate drugs, infections, fever and alcohol withdrawal. The best course of action is to treat the cause of the confusion. Often psychotropic drugs will be required, either benzodiazepines or antipsychotic drugs at a low dose. Try to get advice on management from the most appropriate source, such as the medical staff attached to your team. Dissociative disorders tend to be a response to severe stress and have perplexing presentations. Staff may think that people are having them on, because they may have amnesia or odd neurological signs. They can also appear indifferent to their surroundings and even forget who they are. This is very rare and tends to settle spontaneously.

How to communicate

It is a skill to appear as if you have plenty of time to chat when in fact there is little time to spare. Most people are excellent at talking to people, yet often feel anxious about touching on things that might be upsetting. It is important to overcome this fear and address issues with which people really struggle. This section is little more than a few 'top tips' to help you broach difficult subjects. It is most certainly not an exhaustive list or a recipe for good communication.

People are generally very good communicators. We spend our whole lives in conversations of one sort or other. People evaluate the most subtle of clues and know if you are asking a question but do not really want an answer. It is shown in tiny moves away and eye contact. Saying 'let's talk about you' as you open the door to go is never going to get people to talk. It is very important to state here that there are times when you will not feel able to take on the burdens of others. On those occasions act kindly and, if people start a conversation, ask if you could put it off to the next time. Check that they can manage until then, and when the next time comes you must remember to reinitiate the conversation.

If you want to open a conversation, take a few minutes. Come down to the same level as the person you are talking to, e.g. sit if they are seated. Try not to face them directly because this is quite a challenging posture; you can sit besides them and angle yourself towards them. Unfold your arms and try to appear open and relaxed. Wait a moment.

Try 'We've talked about your cancer; can I ask how you are?'. This is a way to open up the topic that people are more than their cancer. It also implies that the progress of their illness may not reflect their mental state. It may be considered that the cancer has been eradicated, so life expectancy now returns to 'normal', and yet people can be falling apart. Conversely, the cancer may be ravaging the body and yet the person may be peaceful and steady. An alternative is 'I just want to check how you are doing with all of this going on' or 'How are things with your family/wife/husband?'. Or a reasonably neutral question that can open a can of worms: 'I hope you don't mind my asking, but you seem upset.' Often the most valuable thing is just to listen without any pretence that you can change anything. Acknowledging how people feel is such a powerful thing, giving people permission to own their feelings. Again, it suggests that people are more than their feelings.

If you want to explore people's worries in order to offer reassurance, you can try a rather oblique approach, e.g. 'Some people worry about needing a colostomy bag and how they will cope. Do you have any of those concerns?'; or 'People can find it difficult to say they worry about their sexual function after surgery. What do you think?'; or on another tack: 'You seem to be angry.' Anger is very easy to approach – there is a feeling that anger will be directed towards the enquirer, but this rarely happens. Simply noting that the person seems angry is generally enough to defuse things sufficiently to allow discussion: 'Can we talk it through?' Avoid 'squaring up' to the person or mirroring their body language, which can inflame things. Try to keep relaxed, maintain the same open posture, partly facing the person. Note things that are relevant, such as perceived failure of care. Try to address these issues and discuss them with relevant colleagues. Do not allow yourself to be threatened. Say 'I will have to end this conversation because I feel threatened', and then leave the room. Or say 'I want to talk this over with you, but not when you are so angry. Can we talk later when you are calm?'. Stick to the arrangements you have made but first ensure your safety, take a colleague and meet in a neutral place.

Staff stress and how to avoid it

Of course the most important, most fundamental issue is staying well yourself. Little teaching is given on this and many units are full of stressed-out staff (Ramirez et al., 1996). How to avoid getting stressed out is not so easy to answer. In fact, although there is some evidence for the use of staff support groups (Roberts, 1997), these are not relevant for many healthcare professionals, e.g. if you are the only person to hold a position in an area.

Tips to stay well

Things that are important include: doing a job you enjoy; not taking on more than you can manage; telling your boss if things are too busy; and trying to find strategies to cope when things are hectic. Perhaps the most important issue is to be wary of confusing work with life. Be very clear. 'I will only work 9 to 5' or whatever is reasonable. 'I will do my best in that time.' 'My working too hard will not sort out everyone who needs my care.' 'If I let myself get too stressed then I am not giving good care.' Leave work at work and do things you love outside of that time – things for which you are full of passion and that renew you. Take all your holidays. Discuss difficulties with a colleague who can advise you in confidence. Perhaps even find a regular time to go over tough issues with someone you trust, such as a supervisor. Running yourself into the ground serves no end at all. Get appropriate training, e.g. in communication skills.

Tips to get well

If you are stressed, do something about it – do not wait, do not delay. If it is too much, stop doing it. Take some holiday, take some sick leave, get some breathing space. Do not fool yourself into thinking that life is easier on the next rung up the ladder. It rarely is; every rung has its own pressures and responsibilities. Learn how to be happy on your own rung. Look at what has happened and make a plan to avoid a repeat. Be vicious with your time and do not give in. Protect yourself diligently. Take your time. Learn skills such as meditation or yoga. Exercise, eat well, see your mates, invest in your family and enjoy your life because you only get one go. Celebrate a job well done and cut yourself some slack. Do not be hard on yourself – there are plenty of others to do that. Learn how to enjoy it all again. Chat and laugh. Remember that ups and downs are normal; learn how to stop the downs flattening you. Experiment with your life, break your routine, seek out and enjoy surprises, do things 'just to see what happens' and savour it all.

Conclusion

Exploring the impact cancer has on the individual is taxing but enjoyable work. It is part of caring for people who have cancer, alongside the physical care. Cancer can defeat the patient and the professional. Not only does it shorten lives, it can also numb the hearts and minds of everyone involved. To try to avoid this; engage in a dialogue of life. Talk to people about their lives and care for your own. Point to a healthy way to live with cancer and eventually a good way to die. To do this, a professional needs to be healthy. Learn how to care for and refresh yourself. Get involved in your own life; be concerned for others, fresh and alive. We all fall short of this. Yet, I am often struck by how much our smallest words and actions mean to people, how grateful and gracious people are, and how much I still have to learn.

References

Cain E, Kohorn E, Quinlan D, Latimer K, Schwartz P (1986) Psychological benefits of a cancer support group. Cancer 57: 183–189.

Derogatis L, Morrow G, Fetting J (1983) The prevalence of psychiatric disorder amongst cancer patients. Journal of the American Medical Association 249: 751–757.

Garssen B, Goodkin K (1999) On the role of immunological factors as mediators between psychological factors and cancer progression. Psychiatry Research 85(1): 51–61.

Holmes T (1978) Life situations, emotions and disease. Psychosomatic Medicine 19: 747.

Kiecolt-Glaser J, Page G, Marucha P, MacCallum R, Glaser R (1998) Psychological influences on surgical recovery: Perspectives from psychoneuroimmunology. American Psychologist 53: 1209–1218.

Levy J (1997) How does basic research in cancer and AIDS approach the concern for quality of life? In: Cancer AIDS and Quality of Life. New York: Plenum Press, pp. 17–35.

Ramirez A, Graham J, Richards M, Cull A, Gregory W (1996) Mental health of hospital consultants: the effects of stress and satisfaction at work. The Lancet 347: 724–728.

Roberts G (1997) Prevention of burn out. Advances in Psychiatric Treatment 3: 282–289.

World Health Organization (1994) International Classification of Diseases, 10th revision (ICD-10). Geneva: WHO.

Zigmond A, Snaith R (1983) The Hospital Anxiety and Depression Scale. Acta Psychiatrica Scandinavica 67: 361–370.

Further reading

Communication

Brewin T with Sparshott M (1996) Relating to the Relatives. Breaking bad news, communication and support. Oxford: Radcliffe Medical Press Ltd.

Buckman R. (1992) How to Break Bad News. A guide for health care professionals. London: Pan Books.

Stress and some ways to take care of yourself

Firth-Cozens J, Payne R (1999) Stress in Health Professionals. Psychological and organisational causes and interventions. Chichester: John Wiley & Sons Ltd.

Gilbert P (1997) Overcoming Depression. A self-help guide using cognitive behavioural techniques. London: Robinson Publishing Ltd.

Mental illness

Bloch S, Singh BS (1997) Understanding Troubled Minds. A guide to mental illness and its treatment. Melbourne: Melbourne University Press.

CHAPTER 3

The impact of cancer on the family

LINDA KRISTJANSON

Picture a free-floating mobile, each part separate, yet connected by a thread that unifies the whole. Some parts are dancing quickly, propelled by a passing breeze, while other pieces sit relatively quietly, balancing the counterparts as the mobile hangs suspended in the air. The mobile is balanced, interesting, changing and colourful. Then something hits one of the suspended parts. The balance of the mobile is disrupted, the pieces swing wildly and the mobile struggles to restore its equilibrium (Allmond et al., 1979).

The mobile is a useful metaphor when we think of the impact of cancer on the family. When an individual family member is diagnosed with cancer, the family is temporarily thrown off-balance as different members struggle to adapt to the changes, the new roles they might play and a different sense of the future. For some families, members may even experience uncertainty about the stability of the family as a unit in the face of such a threat. Disorder and confusion may occur. Some family members will experience more disruption in their lives than others, but no-one is unaffected by the event. Unlike an episodic short gust of wind that temporarily throws the mobile off-balance, the illness of cancer may, however, continue to pressurize the individual, placing strain on the family together with the need for adaptation. The family continues to be tossed about by the demands of the illness and the often unrelenting pressures that must be faced. The role of the healthcare team, and in particular the nurse, becomes central in assisting families to maintain their balance as they encounter the challenges of cancer and in helping them move forward with some assurance in the family's altered form.

Gastrointestinal cancers pose particular challenges to family members. The overall aim of this chapter is to describe the impact of cancer on the family, with a particular focus on the needs of families of those individuals diagnosed with gastro-intestinal cancer. This chapter discusses how nurses might help families attain some measure of balance and health amidst the challenges of the cancer event. A clinical case example is referred to throughout the chapter to illustrate the points discussed.

Defining the family

Discussions about caring for families require clarification about what is meant by the term 'family'. Families are made up of different individuals who may or may not be related through blood or legal ties. They may include a small one-couple pair, or be made up of a large network of relatives, close friends and neighbours. Families have their own unique biographies, which are shaped by the backgrounds, links, choices and values that they knit together to define themselves as a family unit. Individuals within families will have various needs, commitments, personal histories, personal resources and goals. Therefore, arriving at one agreed-upon definition of a family is difficult to achieve. From a clinical perspective, the most functional approach to defining and knowing the family affected by an illness such as cancer is to allow the patient and his or her family members to self-define the family, so that the unique structure and dynamics of the family can be acknowledged. Failure to recognize the unique nature of families can disenfranchise some family members or lead to simplistic assumptions about who constitutes the family. This is particularly so if families do not fit a stereotypical definition of family (i.e. couple with two children). Individuals who are in homosexual relationships, blended families, families who live geographically apart, and those without apparent formal ties may be neglected in the family care approach if their relationship to the patient is not understood and respected (Kristjanson and Ashcroft, 1994; Leis et al., 1997).

The family as a system

Family systems theory is useful in understanding the impact of an illness such as cancer on the family. It specifies that the members of a family make up the family system and that a change in one part of the family system changes the rest of the system (Bogdan, 1984; Kemp, 1995). The boundaries around the family system vary in their degree of permeability, with some families having rigid and closed boundaries whereas others might be quite open and diffuse. Either end of the extremes of this boundary continuum can be unhealthy – with families who have very rigid boundaries functioning in an isolated and non-adaptive manner, allowing little individuality within the family and being resistant to new information and ideas. At the other extreme of the continuum are families whose boundaries are so diffuse that the family appears to have little identity; they function chaotically, with little sense of connection among members. Families who are able to support each other and allow individuals to express their own forms of individuality while still maintaining a sense of connection to each other are better able to adapt to changes that impinge on the family system (Leis et al., 1997; Wright and Leahy, 1984).

Impact of cancer on the family

The family, not merely the patient, experiences the crisis, long-term effects and consequences of cancer (Northouse and Golden-Peters, 1993; Kristjanson and Ashcroft, 1994). Family members are placed in the position of supporting the patient, physically and emotionally, and serve as a reference point for helping the patient to make meaning out of this event (McLaughlan, 1990; Kristjanson and Ashcroft, 1994). The research undertaken to examine the impact of cancer on the family can be summarized into four key issues which are given in Table 3.1.

Table 3.1 Type of impact on family

Type of impact	Indicators of family distress
Emotional pain	Catastrophic meaning of the event Feelings of loss/threatened loss Isolation
Family communication strains	Protection and gate-keeping Sexuality questions Financial concerns
Information vacuum	Language and volume of information Non-verbal communication Power imbalances Time and space limits
Physical care pressures	Strains and fatigue of the carer role Lack of constancy Role constriction

Emotional pain

The emotional impact of a diagnosis of cancer on the family has been well documented (Northouse and Northouse, 1988; Gotcher, 1992; Kristjanson et al., 1996). Three central emotional processes are usually triggered: questions about the meaning of the event, feelings of loss or threatened loss, and a sense of isolation.

Questions about the meaning of the event

Cancer touches basic aspects of an individual's orientation to living: time, purpose, inclusion and sense of future. The diagnosis of cancer is decidedly an unwelcome event which is not part of the normal expectations of the family's life course. It is all-encompassing, at least for a period of time, and usually takes centre stage in capturing the patient's or family members' energies. Family members will re-examine their views about the future, the quality of their relationships and the choices they have made up to the time of diagnosis. They may search for an explanation for the diagnosis (e.g. diet, environmental risks and hereditary factors), causing them to question, search and struggle for a way of 'making sense' of this event in their lives (Chekryn, 1984). Family members may seek to find someone or something to 'blame' for the disease (e.g. delayed diagnosis, poor self-care on the part of the patient). Sometimes they may blame themselves if they feel that they did not encourage the patient to seek medical attention earlier. These questions can foster guilt, tension, anger and distrust, and make it difficult for family members to support each other and receive support from external sources.

Some family members may begin a positive search for meaning, as they try to augment the closeness of family relationships to help them cope. Family members may reinvest in their relationships in a more committed and compassionate manner and realign their personal goals to allow them to focus more on the patient and the illness situation. The challenge for nurses is to listen carefully for the meaning of the event that family members may create in response to the illness. Sensitive attention to the various questions and fears that may surface in response to this search for meaning will allow the nurse to provide information and reassurance that will help them to interpret the cancer event. A non-defensive, non-judgemental approach in response to family behaviours and emotional reactions is advised, so that the deeper concerns of the families can be heard and understood.

Feelings of loss/threatened loss

The crisis of cancer in the family prompts feelings of loss or threatened loss. These feelings of loss may stem from fears of losing a significant person in their lives and a sense of loss about the hopes and plans that may no longer appear feasible. Family members themselves may become aware of death as a more concrete possibility and consequently may face issues about their own life, such as the choices made or not made and questions about the quality of relationships. A family member may become aware of a sense of aloneness in the world as he or she is brought abruptly face to face with the finite temporal dimension of life.

Isolation

Isolation for the family may occur when friends and other family members do not respond with their physical or emotional presence. Isolation may also occur when some family members must take on most of the care responsibility whereas others withdraw or indicate no understanding of the magnitude of the pain or the process of caring for a loved one. Thus, isolation can take the form of physical, psychological or spiritual absence of others. One of the most isolating situations is when others seek to comfort through inappropriate cheer or inappropriate words by trying to transform bad into good or pain into privilege (Kushner, 1981).

To illustrate the impact of a cancer diagnosis on the family and to describe strategies that nurses can use to help these families, use is made of the story of Pam and Tom:

> Pam was a 53-year-old woman who was diagnosed with cancer of the colon. After surgery she and her husband were informed by the surgeon that her cancer was cured. Pam was a part-time secretary. She had been married to Tom for 28 years. They had two adult children who had demanding careers and they no longer lived at home. Tom was employed as a mechanic and had worked for the same firm for 15 years. Pam resigned from her job as a secretary when her cancer was diagnosed.

The primary care issue for this couple was the initial impact of the diagnosis. The particular meaning for Tom of this news is outlined in Table 3.2 and the nursing strategies used to address these concerns are listed there.

Table 3.2 Initial diagnosis of cancer – case application

Issue	Meaning for family	Nursing strategies
Initial diagnosis of cancer	Uncertainty about the future	Developed rapport with the family Assessed family functioning and resources
	Fear of suffering	Offered reassurance about medical/ nursing knowledge to manage suffering
	Uncertainty about ability to cope	Provided information about available resources to assist with care as needed
	Financial concerns	Used available resources (e.g. social work, cancer support agencies)

Family communication strains

Poor communication causes more suffering to cancer patients and their families than any other problems, with the exception of unrelieved pain (Stedeford, 1981). Communication is essential to healthy family functioning, and families who have limited communication skills are less able to manage stressful situations (Kemp, 1995; Kristjanson et al., 1996). The family's previous patterns of communication determine, to a large extent, the degree of communication that occurs within the family at the time of the cancer. Some family members may be open and clear in their exchanges about the illness, treatment decisions, fears and doubts. Others may be reserved in their expressions of feelings, holding back worries, regrets and uncertainties. These family communication strains may be most apparent in three domains: protection and gate-keeping, sexuality questions and financial concerns.

Protection and gate-keeping

Relationship strains may occur as both the patient and family members endeavour to protect each other from worries and concerns about the illness. Patients may serve as a type of gate-keeper of information, because it is usually the patient who has primary contact with the healthcare team. This is particularly common when parents have cancer and are cautious about sharing information of their illness with their children (Asch-Goodkin, 1994; Nelson et al., 1994). Family members often rely on the patient to convey important information about the illness to help them to know how to cope with the treatment or subsequent phases of the disease, and may feel uncertain or frustrated if they lack information. These protective approaches to communication can contribute to conflict, anxiety and poor communication within the family.

Another communication difficulty can occur if family members become over-protective and infer that the individual is less capable because he or she has a serious illness. This tendency to infer one type of limitation from another is described as 'spread' (Wright, 1960). In the mind of the family member, the patient's limitations spread from one domain to another. For example, if the family member observes that the patient has a physical limitation (e.g. difficulty moving independently), the family member may transfer this view of the patient's deficit from a physical one to a mental, cognitive or verbal deficit. They may then offer more assistance than is needed or offer assistance in domains that are not necessary (e.g. answering for the patient, making decisions that he or she is capable of making). This protective response may be well intended, but can create barriers and conflict within the family.

Sexuality questions

Issues related to sexuality are relevant to both the early diagnostic and later stages of the cancer experience. Literature related to sexual changes caused by a cancer illness is inconsistent. Some studies report that couples experience an enhanced closeness and satisfaction with their sexual relationships (Nishimoto, 1995). Other research documents incongruent perceptions of sexual satisfaction between patients and partners (Burt, 1995; Monga et al., 1997). Issues of intimacy, closeness and sexual interactions are not always clearly distinguished in these studies, clouding interpretations of the findings.

Partners of patients who have a colostomy may be uncertain about how to maintain a physical relationship with the patient (Kluka and Kristjanson, 1996). The patient may experience embarrassment or changes to self-image that affect the couple's relationship. These issues may receive little attention because they are not life threatening. However, issues of sexuality can have a significant impact on the well-being of the patient and family. Few individuals have an opportunity to discuss their concerns about sexuality because it is perceived as a relatively unimportant topic and a highly personal subject. As sexual desire is a private matter for most people, a consequence of that privacy is that there is little opportunity for individuals to develop an objective perspective about their experiences. Thus, most people are left alone with their thoughts, feelings, desires and impulses. There are few opportunities to speak about these concerns to others, and even fewer chances of finding good advice when actions are in doubt. Apart from making themselves available to listen objectively to others' sexual problems, nurses can help locate pertinent information among the range of self-help and other books available on the subject of sexuality. In addition, people who struggle with sexual feelings nearly always respond positively to the opportunity to talk about their struggles (Kemp, 1995; Nishimoto, 1995).

Financial concerns

Given et al. (1994) have documented the financial concerns that family members experience when a member has an illness such as cancer. Children in the family, spouses and other dependent members may share these worries (Asch-Goodkin, 1994; Nelson et al., 1994). Costs of care may be an issue, e.g. family members may worry about the ongoing costs of medications and treatment. Indirect costs associated with providing care or taking time off work to attend appointments or provide assistance to the patient may also be a source of concern (Chochinov and Kristjanson, 1998). Family members may be reluctant to disclose these concerns, or feel guilty about having worries about financial matters when the patient is so ill and may be suffering. Family members who are preoccupied with financial concerns may be distracted and less able to give attention to the patient's care needs (Kristjanson et al., 1998). A simple question about how families might be coping with the financial changes or pressures as a consequence of the illness may elicit these fears and allow nurses to make appropriate referrals or help family members identify resources to help them to manage. The opportunity to discuss these concerns may also ease the strain for family members who may be reluctant to discuss these matters with the patient or others.

Six months after the surgery Pam presented to hospital with nausea, vomiting and abdominal pain. She was diagnosed with a bowel obstruction from widespread tumour recurrence and was found to have metastases to her liver. Both Tom and Pam were devastated by this news, angry with the healthcare team and no longer trusting of them. The surgeon offered Pam the choice of further surgery or conservative management of the obstruction. Pam was also referred to an oncologist. Pam refused any further treatment although Tom wanted her to consider all treatment options available. Tom was angry with Pam for her decision not to proceed with treatment, but the children fully supported their mother's decision. Tom continued to work while Pam was in hospital and was only able to visit in the evenings. This made it difficult for him to obtain information about her condition and care. When Tom was able to speak to staff he was given conflicting information from different members of the team.

Family care issues, the meaning of these events for Tom and nursing strategies used to address these concerns are shown in Table 3.3.

Table 3.3 Family communication issues – case application

Issues	Meaning for family	Nursing strategies
Lack of trust in the healthcare team	Feelings of fear and isolation	Developed a supportive relationship with Tom Assessed the cause of his mistrust Acknowledged and accepted his sense of mistrust Ensured that the healthcare team were aware of situation Used open empathetic communication
Relationship strain and conflict within the family related to treatment options	Lack of control Poor family communication Anger Frustration Isolation	Acknowledged Tom's difficult situation Provided support Provided information about options Encouraged family communication Initiated family meeting to facilitate open discussion
Poor communication between the healthcare team and Tom	Lack of accurate information Confusion Isolation	Allowed time to communicate with Tom when visiting Assessed Tom's information needs Ensured adequate communication among members of the healthcare team Helped to identify plan of care for Pam with Pam and the family through use of a family meeting

Information vacuum

The literature consistently documents difficulties that family members of cancer patients report about access to information (Northouse and Northouse, 1988; Hileman et al., 1992; Kristjanson and Ashcroft, 1994; Kluka and Kristjanson, 1996). These difficulties are described in four ways: difficulties with the language and volume of information, the meaning placed on non-verbal communication exchanges, power imbalances, and time and space limitations for information exchange.

Language and volume difficulties

Family members describe difficulties obtaining specific, straightforward information in a format that they can understand. Use of medical jargon is frequently mentioned as a barrier to adequate communication about the plan of care (Northouse and Northouse, 1988; McLaughlan, 1990). Language barriers may also be a problem if patients and family members do not share the same language and cultural background as the healthcare professional (McLaughlan, 1990; McNamara et al., 1999). In addition, differences in educational levels between health professionals and patients/families can create problems with exchange of content (Mor et al., 1992).

Health professionals may overload family members with large amounts of information or may provide information in small amounts in an effort not to overwhelm them with too much detail. This can create difficulties because family members vary in their ways of assimilating and integrating information (Northouse and Northouse, 1988; Kristjanson, 2000).

Non-verbal communication

About 80% of communication may occur at a non-verbal level, making this aspect of communication extremely important (Gotcher, 1992). Non-verbal communication may convey substantial messages that override verbal statements. A healthcare professional who appears worried or avoids eye contact may communicate to the patient and family that he or she is discouraged about the plan of care and not optimistic about the patient's ability to cope with the illness. Healthcare providers who are abrupt, unusually cheerful or patronizing in their tone of voice may also create communication barriers (Kristjanson, 2000).

Power imbalances

An equal and balanced relationship exchange implies that both parties are able to share information, ask questions, and convey emotions and reactions in an open and authentic manner. If this view of the patient–health professional relationship does not exist, it is more likely that one will be allocated the role of imparting information and asking questions, with the other responding in a more passive, reactive manner (Kristjanson, 2000). Relationship issues associated with communication are particularly problematic when health professionals are insensitive to the imbalance in power and control that patients and families may feel. Family members report a hesitancy to bother busy health professionals with questions about care because they believe that the healthcare providers are primarily responsible to the patient and that their needs and concerns are tangential (Northouse and Northouse, 1988). Therefore, efforts by healthcare providers to reach out to families are important.

Time and space limitations

The importance of communication with the family is partly represented by the time and space created or allotted for this communication exchange. The apparent lack of space for discussion about care plans and goals conveys a message that this interchange is not very important. It is not unusual for patients and families to report communication about treatment and care in the hallways of busy hospitals, over the phone or in small clinic rooms, with little privacy or time for discussion (Mor et al, 1992; Kristjanson, 2000). Health professionals may also limit their information sharing with patients and families because of the pace of their busy work schedules, an assumption that the patient/family has understood the information conveyed, and a lack of comfort in knowing how to communicate difficult/bad news (McLaughlan, 1990; Bottorff et al., 1995).

Attention to the factors that limit effective communication exchanges between family members and healthcare providers may assist families to fill this information vacuum and feel more confident about coping with the patient's illness. Families who are well informed are able to function in a supportive role and experience less illness-related anxiety (Taylor et al., 1993; Kristjanson et al., 1998).

Pam's condition deteriorated and she entered the terminal phase of her illness. Symptoms of pain and nausea were well controlled. She also developed symptoms of weakness and anorexia. Tom was extremely concerned about her lack of nutrition and insisted on ordering meals for her, attempting to feed her against her wishes. As Pam's condition deteriorated further she was unable to swallow and Tom recognized that she had no oral intake at all and requested that intravenous fluids be commenced.

Information care issues confronting this family and nursing strategies used to address these issues are shown in Table 3.4.

Table 3.4 Information needs – case application

Issues	Meaning for family	Nursing strategies
Nutrition	Lack of control Need for Tom to be 'doing something' Fear that Pam will starve to death Reality that Pam is dying	Acknowledged Tom's distress Provided information about food in the terminal stages (i.e. decreased need for food, effect of food on increasing nausea, issue of dysphagia) Encouraged Tom to assist with other aspects of care
Hydration	Assumption that Pam is not receiving care Belief that 'fluids maintain life' Belief that lack of fluids will cause Pam discomfort Belief that lack of fluids will cause death	Acknowledged Tom's distress Emphasize that sensitive and attentive care is being given Provided information to Tom about the benefits of dehydration (i.e. decreased pulmonary secretions, less vomiting, less pain, less oedema)
	Need for Tom to be 'doing something'	Encourage Tom to provide mouth care and assist with other aspects of care

Physical care pressures

Family caregiving demands may be substantial when a patient is confronted with a cancer diagnosis. Family members may need to assume duties that the ill person cannot undertake, and may experience practical problems associated with transportation to treatments, management of child care, unrelenting work demands that do not take the patient's illness into consideration, and challenges of maintaining a normal functioning household. A number of factors make these pressures more difficult: role strain and carer fatigue, lack of constancy and role constriction.

Strains and fatigue of the carer role

Family members perform roles in relation to each other, based on expectations of what each person should do. These roles shift and change during the course of a lifetime, but generally family members have a script in their minds about how each person's role in the family will be played. When one person's ability to perform his or her role changes (as in the case of illness), the script no longer fits and the other people in the family must undergo reciprocal role changes. The assumption of new roles may be stressful as family members learn or accept new parts. Some may welcome the chance to take on a role as carer or decision-maker. However, often the negotiation and shift of new roles take time and the transition for all family members and the individual may be awkward.

Pressures on family carers are also associated with the composition of the family, e.g. families with few members, those with young children and families who are isolated may be particularly burdened by physical caring tasks because there are fewer individuals with whom to share the load. As cancer is a disease of elderly people, family members may also be older and have their own health problems (Brody and Lang, 1982; Cobbs, 1998). These additional stresses may make physical caregiving and the assumption of extra practical tasks more difficult or impossible.

Family members often experience carer fatigue (Jensen and Given, 1991). The assumptions of new roles may have been gradual and their feelings of responsibility for care of the ill person may prevent them from seeing alternative ways of receiving help with care. Families may require help to problem-solve the demands created by the illness (Given and Given, 1998). This problem-solving might begin by helping family members to recognize that their own health must also be maintained if they are to offer support to the patient. Instances of deterioration of the family carer's health while caring for an ill member are not uncommon (Kristjanson and Ashcroft, 1994; Given and Given, 1998). Carer fatigue may occur because carers are unaware of the availability of resources that could be called upon to decrease the strain on the family. Some may experience fatigue because there is an underlying feeling of duty or guilt that is satisfied through an endless devotion to caring. Carer fatigue is not limited to small isolated families. Family carers who are members of large families can experience this fatigue as well because one person may be singled out as the primary carer.

Lack of constancy

The lack of constancy in the ill person's functional abilities may also pose difficulties. The illness may have a steady downward progression, resulting in gradual decreases in the patient's ability to fulfil various roles and duties. The family must then recognize subtle changes in the individual's condition and gradually assume more tasks that the person is unable to perform. On the other hand, illness may be characterized by exacerbations and remissions, necessitating episodic changes in the person's ability to perform roles. At times, the sick role may fit more appropriately and at other times the patient may feel healthy and able to take on more tasks and responsibilities within the family. Change, even when it involves improvement, adds stress (Edwards and Cooper, 1988; Spector, 1997). The constant fluidity and adaptation of roles in these instances requires much work and negotiation on the part of the family. Individuals within the family may also have different perceptions of the individual's illness and the extent to which his or her competence is affected. In addition, an uncertain time trajectory for the illness may make the demands more difficult, because family members are unsure of how long they may be required to undertake the additional physical tasks, limiting their abilities to pace their energies.

Role constriction

Family members may also experience role constriction when the carer eliminates other previously held social roles and takes on only one role – that of caregiver. The result can be a kind of 'cabin fever', which develops gradually and can impact on the carer's health. Family members may need help to identify how much constriction they will tolerate. Families may need help to consider the patient's level of disability and dependence, their own health, their other responsibilities and roles, and the availability of other assistance. Families with rigid boundaries and a strong sense of caregiving duty may be most resistant to external help and may need encouragement to accept resources.

> Physical care pressures became a factor when a decision arose about where Pam should die. Tom and Pam's children wanted Pam to die at home. Tom felt unable to cope with Pam's physical care at home. Pam was admitted to the Hospice and died peacefully with her family present.

This issue and nursing care approaches used to address this concern are outlined in Table 3.5.

Table 3.5 Physical care pressures – case application

Issues	Meaning for family	Nursing strategies
Place of care	Feeling pressured to make the 'correct' decision about place of care (i.e. hospital, hospice, home) Feeling inadequate and that he is letting his family down by not being able to care for Pam at home	Informed family of all options in relation to terminal care Supported Tom in his decision Used available resources (e.g. palliative care team, allied health)

In summary, the family care provided to Pam and Tom was challenging and not without error. However, efforts to build trust, support the family and help them to cope with this difficult illness trajectory led to a sense of resolution for the family.

Recommendations for care of families

Approaches to helping families cope with these complicated and challenging issues are not simple and do not apply equally well to all families. However, it is essential that nurses carefully assess the unique needs of families and work with them in an open and supportive manner, in order to identify approaches to care that are suitable for the patient and families (Artinian, 1995; Bottorff et al., 1995). Some general goals of family care and family care strategies can be identified that may be helpful (Table 3.6).

Table 3.6 Goals and strategies to promote health and coping of families

Family care goals	Family care strategies
Family as unit of care	Identification of family members' needs using systematic assessment methods/tools Identify high-risk/high-need families or family members
Communication with family	View family as a source of information Identify clear care goals with family Create space and time for families Communicate within healthcare team so that consistent messages are given to the family

(contd)

Table 3.6 (contd)

Family care goals	Family care strategies
Augment family resources	Identify family resources and strengths Anticipate needs that families may have for their carer roles Educate family members about caregiving duties Identify need for respite/extra support to prevent carer fatigue
High-quality patient care	Provide responsive, individualized care to patient Respect patient's and family's views of patient's needs and symptoms Seek expert consultation when necessary Facilitate communication with patient and family about care needs and plan of care

Healthcare providers who view the family as the unit of care are better able to assess and anticipate the needs of family members and identify those who may be less able to cope. Specific assessment of the needs of individual family members may be particularly helpful when the nurse is attempting to understand the impact of the illness on various members. This early assessment may help the nurse to plan care, anticipate needs, and build trust and rapport with the family (Thorne and Robinson, 1988). Communication with family members is the adhesive that allows good care practices to be realized. Creating time, space and a forum for family discussions and information sharing is central to appropriate family-centred care (Northouse and Golden-Peters, 1993). Family members who are unduly stressed, in conflict with each other or with the healthcare team, and who are poorly informed about how to participate in the care of the patient are less able to help the patient cope with the illness challenges ahead.

References

Allmond BW, Brickman W, Gofman HF (1979) The Family is the Patient. St Louis, MO: CV Mosby Co.

Artinian BM (1995) Risking involvement with cancer patients. Western Journal of Nursing Research 17: 292--304.

Asch-Goodkin J (1994) Children touched by cancer. Contemporary Paediatrics 11(12): 22-26.

Bogdan JL (1984) Family organisation as ecology of ideas: An alternative to the reification of family systems. Family Process 23: 375-388.

Bottorff JL, Gogag M, Engelberg-Lotzkar M (1995) Comforting: Exploring the work of cancer nurses. Journal of Advanced Nursing 22: 1077-1084.

Brody EM, Lang A (1982) 'They can't do it all': aging daughters with aging mothers. Generations 7: 18-20.

Burt K (1995) The effects of cancer on body image and sexuality. Nursing Times 91(7): 36-37.

Chekryn J (1984) Cancer recurrence: Personal meaning, communication and marital adjustment. Cancer Nursing 7: 491-498.

Chochinov HM, Kristjanson LJ (1998) Dying to pay: The cost of end-of-life care. Journal of Palliative Care 14(4): 5-15.

Cobbs EL (1998) Health of older women. Medical Clinical of North America 82: 127-144.

Edwards JR, Cooper CL (1988) The impacts of positive psychological states on physical health: A review and theoretical framework Social Science and Medicine 27: 1447-1459.

Given BA, Given CW (1998) Health promotion for family caregivers of chronically ill elders. Annual Review of Nursing Research 16: 197-217.

Given BA, Given GW, Stommel M (1994) Family and out-of-pocket costs for women with breast cancer. Cancer Practice: A Multidisciplinary Journal of Cancer Care 2: 189-193.

Gotcher JM (1992) Interpersonal communication and psychosocial adjustment. Journal of Psychosocial Oncology 10(3): 21-39.

Hileman J, Lackey N, Hassanein R (1992) Identifying the needs of home caregivers of patients with cancer. Oncology Nursing Forum 19: 771-777.

Jensen S, Given BA (1991) Fatigue affecting family caregivers of cancer patients. Cancer Nursing 14: 181-187.

Kemp C (1995) Terminal Illness: A guide to nursing care. Toronto: JB Lippincott Co.

Kluka S, Kristjanson LJ (1996) Development and testing of the Ostomy Concerns (OC) Scale: Measuring concerns of ostomy cancer patients and spouses (OC) scale. Journal of Enterostomal Therapy (3): 166-170.

Kristjanson LJ (2000) Establishing goals of care: communication traps and treatment lane changes. In: Ferrell B, Coyle N (eds), Palliative Care Nursing. Oxford: Oxford University Press, pp. 331-338.

Kristjanson LJ, Ashcroft T (1994) The family's cancer journey: A literature review. Cancer Nursing 17(1): 1-17.

Kristjanson LJ, Sloan JA, Dudgeon DJ, Adaskin E (1996) Family members' perceptions of palliative cancer care: Predictors of family functioning and family members' health. Journal of Palliative Care 12(4): 10-20.

Kristjanson LJ, Nikoletti S, Porock D, Smith M, Lobchuk M, Pedler P (1998) Congruence between patients' and family caregivers' perceptions of symptom distress in patients with terminal cancer. Journal of Palliative Care 14(1): 24-32.

Kushner HS (1981) When Bad Things Happen to Good People. New York: Avon.

Leis A, Kristjanson LJ, Koop P, Laizner A (1997) Family health and the palliative care trajectory: A research agenda. Canadian Journal of Clinical Oncology 1: 352-360.

McLaughlan CAJ (1990) Handling distressed relatives and breaking bad news. British Medical Journal 301:1145-1149.

McNamara B, Martin K, Waddell C, Yuen K (1999) Palliative care in a multicultural society: Perceptions of health care providers. Palliative Medicine 11: 359–367.

Monga U, Tan G, Ostermann HJ, Monga TN (1997) Sexuality in head and neck cancer patients. Archives of Physical Medicine and Rehabilitation 78: 298–304.

Mor V, Masterson-Allen S, Houts P (1992) The changing needs of patients with cancer at home: A longitudinal view. Cancer 69: 829–838.

Nelson E, Sloper P, Charlton A, White D (1994) Children who have a parent with cancer: A pilot study Journal of Cancer Education 9(1): 30–36.

Nishimoto PW (1995) Sex and sexuality in the cancer patient. Nurse Practitioner Forum 6: 221–227.

Northouse LL, Golden-Peters H (1993) Cancer and the family: Strategies to assist spouses. Seminars in Oncology Nursing 9(2): 74–82.

Northouse PG, Northouse LL (1988) Communication and cancer: Issues confronting patients, health professionals, and family members. Journal of Psychosocial Oncology 5(3): 17–45.

Spector NH (1997) The great Hans Selye and the great 'stress' muddle. Developmental Brain Dysfunction 10: 538–542.

Stedeford A (1981) Couples facing death: Unsatisfactory communication. British Medical Journal ii: 1098.

Taylor EJ, Ferrell BR, Grant M, Cheyney L (1993) Managing cancer pain at home: The decisions and ethical conflicts of patients, family caregivers, and homecare nurses. Oncology Nursing Forum 20: 919–927.

Thorne SE, Robinson CA (1988) Reciprocal trust in health care relationships. Journal of Advanced Nursing 13: 782–789.

Wright B (1960) Physical Disability: A psychological approach. New York: Harper & Row.

Wright L, Leahy M (1984) Nurses and Families: A guide to family assessment and intervention. Philadelphia: FA Davis Co.

CHAPTER 4

Cancer of the upper aerodigestive tract: head and neck

PETER RHYS EVANS AND FRAN RHYS EVANS

Head and neck cancer accounts for only 10% of malignant tumours and yet nowhere else in the gastrointestinal tract are the effects of progression of disease more readily apparent, more cosmetically deforming, and more functionally and psychologically disturbing than in this region. Basic functions such as breathing, eating, speech, hearing and sight, as well as the patient's appearance, may be dramatically altered and with such changes comes the emotional trauma of reintegration back into society.

It is essential that nurses involved in this demanding speciality have a sound theoretical knowledge of the anatomy and physiology of the region, the disease process and the various treatment options. Surgery often involves complex reconstructive procedures for single-stage restoration of function and appearance, and the rehabilitation process requires comprehensive support from various members of the multidisciplinary team (Table 4.1).

Incidence

Cancer of the upper aerodigestive tract includes a wide range of malignant tumours arising from multiple diverse structures and tissues. The most common site is the larynx but other sites include the lips, the oral cavity and tongue, the pharynx (nasopharynx, oropharynx and hypopharynx), the cervical oesophagus and trachea, and the nasal cavity and sinuses. Tumours of other associated structures such as the thyroid and salivary glands, the ear, orbit and skull base, as well as malignant

Table 4.1 Multidisciplinary care team

Team members
Clinical nurse specialist
Nursing staff
Dietitian
Speech and language therapist
Physiotherapist
Pain management specialist
Pharmacist
Dentist
Dental hygienist
Maxillofacial prosthodontist
Occupational therapist
Community liaison nurse
Social worker
Palliative care team
Chaplain

lumps in the neck, whether caused by metastatic disease or lymphomas, are also an essential part of the scope of head and neck cancer (Table 4.2).

Table 4.2 Number and incidence (%) of head and neck cancers in the UK for 1988

Site	England No. (%)	Scotland No. (%)	Wales No. (%)	N. Ireland No. (%)	UK No. (%)
Larynx	1926 (4.0)	243 (4.7)	155 **(5.4)**	52 (3.3)	2376 (4.2)
Oral cavity (total)	1664 (3.5)	294 **(5.8)**	138 (4.8)	60 (3.8)	2156 3.8)
Lip	243 (0.5)	58 **(1.1)**	24 (0.8)	17 **(1.1)**	342 (0.6)
Mouth	805 (1.7)	158 **(3.1)**	63 (2.2)	27 (1.7)	1053 (1.8)
Tongue	616 (1.3)	78 (1.5)	51 (1.8)	16 (1.0)	761 (1.3)
Pharynx	1006 (1.7)	122 (2.4)	82 **(2.9)**	31 (2.0)	1241 (2.2)
Thyroid	792 (1.7)	99 (1.9)	65 **(2.3)**	23 (1.5)	979 (1.7)
Population (m)	47.4	5.09	2.85	1.57	57.0

Percentage figures in bold represent higher industrial area incidences well above the national average and also higher rural incidence for lip.

There are almost 7000 new head and neck cancers seen annually in the UK with a male:female ratio of 2:1. It affects patients mainly in the sixth and seventh decades and there is a wide regional variation ranging from about 8 per 100 000 population in the south of England to 13–15 per 100 000 in north-west England, Wales and Scotland. Although cancer of individual sites within the head and neck is rare, collectively the combined rate for these tumours represents the eighth most common cancer in males (sixteenth in females) (Rhys Evans and Henk, 2003).

Pathology

The large majority (80%) of tumours are squamous cell carcinomas which arise from the surface mucosa of the upper aerodigestive tract as an ulcerative or exophytic mass (Figure 4.1). They will grow locally, invading adjacent structures, and then usually spread to the draining lymph nodes in the neck where they are confined for some time. The presence of cervical node metastases is the single most adverse prognostic factor in head and neck cancer, reducing survival by a factor of 50%. Only about 10%, however, will eventually metastasize to other organs. Spread to the local nodes depends largely on the effectiveness of lymphatic drainage, with early spread from the nasopharynx, tonsil and tongue base where there are rich lymphatics, and rare neck node involvement from the vocal cords, which are virtually free of lymphatics. Metastases from the breast, lungs and gastrointestinal tract may also appear in the lower neck.

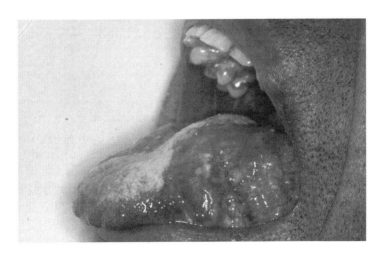

Figure 4.1 Carcinoma of the lateral border of the tongue.

Other tumours include adenocarcinoma, adenoid cystic carcinoma and mucoepidermoid carcinoma, which arise from the major (parotid, submandibular) and minor (oral and nasal cavities, pharynx and larynx) salivary glands, lymphomas which usually present as a rubbery neck swelling and rarely sarcomas. Melanomas arise in the skin as elsewhere, but may also rarely occur as mucosal lesions in the nasal and oral cavities.

Aetiology

Tobacco is by far the most important aetiological factor in head and neck cancer and up to 90% of patients with cancers of the oral cavity, oropharynx, hypopharynx and larynx have used it at some stage. From the Indian subcontinent, the habit of chewing tobacco is especially important in causing oral cancers. Alcohol has an important synergistic effect when combined with tobacco.

Prevention

Cancer of the head and neck is largely a preventable disease and the benefits of eliminating tobacco and reducing alcohol intake are well documented. A well-balanced diet including fruit and vegetables, with supplements of vitamins A, C and E, probably offers some protection. The greatest cost–benefit is gained by educating children not to take up the habit of tobacco use and increasing public awareness of early symptoms. Early detection of small volume disease, particularly in high-risk groups, would significantly improve survival and reduce morbidity associated with extensive surgery.

Clinical presentation

Inflammatory conditions of the head and neck are very common, but invariably resolve spontaneously or with a course of antibiotics. Any symptoms such as hoarseness, difficulty with swallowing, a sore throat, or a lump in the neck or ulcer in the mouth that persists for more than 2–3 weeks should be considered a result of cancer until proved otherwise. The level of suspicion should be further increased if there is a history of smoking or heavy alcohol intake, particularly if the patient is aged over 45 years, or if there are two or more symptoms. Persistent pain at any site is an indication of advanced disease. A list of the common symptoms is given in Table 4.3.

Table 4.3 Common head and neck cancer symptoms

Presenting symptom	Suspicious site (%)
Hoarseness	Larynx (80–90)
	Hypopharynx (50)
Neck lump	Oropharynx and nasopharynx (80–90)
	Hypopharynx (50)
	Thyroid (90)
Sore throat/dysphagia	Hypopharynx and oropharynx (80–90)
	Larynx (30–40)
Earache	Oropharynx, tongue (70–80)
Pain/ulceration/visible lesion	Oral cavity, tongue (80–90)
Unilateral deafness	Nasopharynx (50)
Nasal obstruction/bleeding	Nasal cavity/sinuses (80–90)
Lump in parotid/submandibular gland	Salivary gland (90)

Investigations

Head and neck cancer is designated a rare tumour and on aver-age a general ENT (ear, nose and throat) or oral surgeon will see fewer than 10 new cases each year. In line with Government recommendations, all patients should be treated by an appropri-ate multidisciplinary team of head and neck specialists (ENT/head and neck surgeon, maxillofacial surgeon, plastic surgeon, radiotherapist and oncologist), who should see at least 80-100 new patients annually in a cancer unit. This may or may not be part of the local ENT/oral/plastic surgery department and appropriate referral to a member of the team should be made on suspicion or diagnosis of the cancer. It is preferable that investi-gations are carried out by the specialists who will be deciding on and coordinating treatment.

In patients with suspicious ENT symptoms or signs, an initial examination of the appropriate part should be carried out, as well as palpation of the neck to detect any obvious lymphadenopathy (Figure 4.2). Tumours of the oral cavity may be easily visible (see Figure 4.1), but many lesions are difficult to see and a full ENT examination is essential.

Fibreoptic examination carried out in the clinic under local anaesthetic provides a quick and accurate assessment of any lesion in the nasal cavity, pharynx or larynx (Figure 4.3), in addi-tion to general ENT examination. Fine needle aspiration cytology (FNAC) of any swelling in the neck, thyroid or salivary glands should be carried out at the same clinic visit, if appropriate, to

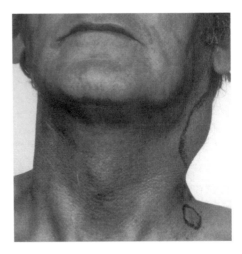

Figure 4.2 Nodal metastases from an apparently occult primary found on investigation to be in the left tonsil.

allow rapid confirmation of diagnosis. Routine haematological tests, a chest radiograph and ECG are carried out to determine the general physical state of the patient, as well as computed tomography (CT) of the head, neck and thorax to assess the extent of the disease and any metastases or second primaries. Additional information may be gained in tumours at some sites with magnetic resonance imaging (MRI). A barium swallow may be helpful in assessment of dysphagia in hypopharyngeal or cervical oesophageal lesions.

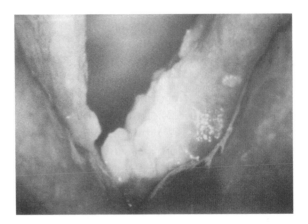

Figure 4.3 Microlaryngoscopy appearance of early vocal cord carcinoma presenting with 3 months of hoarsenesss – cured with radiotherapy.

A pharyngoscopy and microlaryngoscopy under general anaesthetic are then necessary to allow biopsy and assessment of tumour extent, as well as detection of any second primaries.

A special word of caution is required for patients presenting with a suspicious lump in the neck without any obvious upper aerodigestive tract symptoms because many of these will be found on detailed examination to have small squamous cancers of the tonsil or nasopharynx.

Stage and prognosis

The overall 5-year survival rate for head and neck cancers is good (males – 72%; females – 54%) particularly when compared with malignant tumours at other sites. Although there have been great advances in treatment over the past 20 years, notably developments in immediate reconstructive surgery and voice restoration after total laryngectomy, long-term survival has not changed significantly. Restoration of function, quality of life and 3-year survival figures are very much better, but in the longer term other smoking-related diseases (lung cancer, second primaries, heart disease and strokes) take their toll.

The TNM classification is used to designate the stage and extent of the tumour (T) and the presence or absence of nodes (N) and metastases (M). For squamous carcinoma the treatment, prognosis and 5-year survival depend not only on the stage but also on the site of the tumour, as shown in Table 4.4 (Robin et al., 1983). In the UK, the majority (60%) of laryngeal cancers occur on the vocal cords, which have an excellent prognosis (90% for stage I and 80% for stage II) because they present early with persistent hoarseness, and there is poor lymphatic drainage from the cords with the result that node metastases are uncommon. Cancers of the pharynx, on the other hand, have a poor prognosis of 20–40% because of late symptomatic diagnosis and frequent nodal metastases resulting from a rich lymphatic drainage.

The prognosis for malignant salivary gland tumours depends on whether they are high grade (adenoid cystic, squamous cell, high-grade mucoepidermoid and adenocarcinoma) or low grade (acinic cell, low-grade mucoepidermoid and adenocarcinoma) and also on the stage at diagnosis. Rarer tumours such as sarcomas, melanomas and neuroectodermal tumours have an intermediate prognostic outlook, mainly depending on the extent at diagnosis.

Table 4.4 Five-year survival rate for head and neck cancer (percentage – age adjusted) from the West Midlands Cancer Registry

Site	Males	Females
Skin – squamous cell carcinoma	91	86
Skin – melanoma	43	66
Oral cavity	41	45
Oropharynx	19	37
Nasopharynx	25	20
Hypopharynx	12	11
Nasal cavity/sinuses	32	38
Larynx	56	56
Lymphoma	57	57
Sarcoma	37	52
Head and neck overall	72	54

From Robin et al. (1983).

Treatment

The overall national cure rates for cancer treatment in this country are poor (Rhys Evans, 2003) compared with specialist centres in most other Western countries, where cancer is mainly treated by cancer specialists working in specialist cancer centres rather than by general hospital departments. It is therefore essential that head and neck cancers are treated in a specialist unit and it is hoped that results will improve with this centralization of cancer care in the UK.

For head and neck cancer, surgery and radiotherapy, either alone or in combination, are the two main forms of treatment. In early disease, excellent cure rates are usually achievable with either modality used on its own, but for advanced tumours combined therapy with surgery and postoperative radiotherapy are invariably necessary to obtain optimal results. In many situations, however, organ preservation (tongue, larynx) is an important consideration for quality of life and some compromise may have to be made with informed consent between chances of cure and functional preservation.

Treatment of the lymph nodes in the neck (with surgery or radiotherapy depending on the treatment to the primary) is an integral part of management even if no nodes are palpable because of the high risk of occult micrometastases.

Surgery

Surgery offers the most definitive treatment for the majority of cancers of the head and neck, with the purpose of complete excision and immediate reconstruction for larger defects to minimize functional loss. Wide margins of excision are often difficult to achieve because of vital adjacent neurovascular structures such as the carotid artery and cranial nerves, but postoperative radiotherapy will reduce the risk of local recurrence after larger resections.

Advances in reconstructive techniques using pedicle flaps from the chest, and free flaps from the forearm, abdomen, shoulder and small bowel, have allowed effective immediate restoration of function and cosmesis using skin, muscle, fascia, mucosa and bone fashioned appropriately to restore the defect.

Radiotherapy

Radiotherapy is an effective treatment for smaller-volume squamous cancers and for the majority of carcinomas of the tonsil, nasopharynx and lymphomas even with large nodal disease. It has the great advantage of preservation of structural function and is therefore used in most carcinomas of the larynx (see Figure 4.3), and tongue base where the only alternative may be total glossectomy. Unfortunately not all carcinomas are responsive to radiotherapy, particularly larger tumours and lymph node metastases, and salvage surgery is often required for recurrent disease. This is associated with more difficult surgery, a greater risk of complications and poorer outcome. Primary radiotherapy is not advisable for tumours involving bone or cartilage because of the risk of radionecrosis.

Chemotherapy

Chemotherapy is not a curative treatment for squamous carcinomas of the head and neck, and its role is mainly palliative for recurrent or advanced disease not appropriate for curative treatment. There is some evidence that its use together with radiotherapy may improve survival for certain advanced head and neck tumours, but any use should be in the context of prospective clinical trials.

Treatment at specific sites

Oral cavity

Small tumours of the tongue and floor of mouth can be treated with either excision or brachytherapy (radiotherapy implant); larger lesions (see Figure 4.1) are best treated with surgery and reconstruction using a free radial forearm flap with excellent functional results (Figure 4.4). Treatment of the neck is essential except for the small superficial lesions.

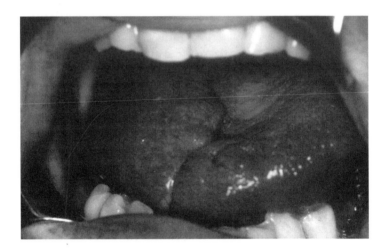

Figure 4.4 Free radial forearm flap for reconstruction after partial glossectomy.

Nasopharynx

All tumours including the neck nodes are treated with radiotherapy with 70–80% locoregional control.

Oropharynx

Functional disturbance of swallowing is a main factor in deciding treatment and many smaller tumours of the tonsil and tongue base will respond to radiotherapy, keeping salvage surgery in reserve for any recurrence. For larger tumours, combined surgery and reconstruction with postoperative radiotherapy gives a better chance of cure.

Hypopharynx and cervical oesophagus

Low cure rates are the result of late presentation and node

metastases. Radiotherapy is effective only for very early tumours and the majority of others (80%) will need pharyngolaryngectomy with stomach 'pull-up' or jejunum free graft reconstruction (Figures 4.5 and 4.6) at some stage. This radical surgery is much more effective if carried out for the primary presentation rather than for recurrence, and most patients can subsequently undergo surgical voice restoration (see below).

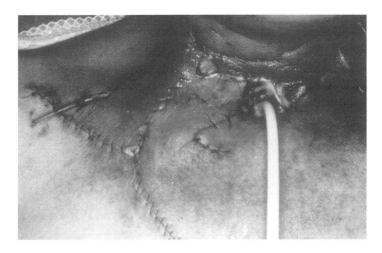

Figure 4.5 Peristomal infection and fistula after pharyngolaryngectomy with free jejunum graft. The Foley catheter is placed through the tracheo-oesophageal voice fistula tract at operation for postoperative feeding. Once oral feeding is established the catheter is removed and replaced with the voice valve (see Figure 4.6).

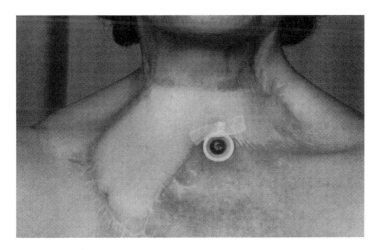

Figure 4.6 Complete healing after 6 months using latissimus dorsi flap. The Blom–Singer speech valve is in place and the patient has an excellent voice.

Larynx

Radiotherapy is effective for most laryngeal cancers except advanced tumours with airway obstruction or cartilage invasion. Partial laryngectomy with avoidance of permanent tracheostomy is possible for early recurrences, but total laryngectomy may be necessary for advanced disease and most recurrences. The functional disability caused by removal of the voice box should, however, be minimized by restoration of near normal voice with a tracheo-oesophageal speech valve, which is now routinely carried out at the time of total laryngectomy (see Figure 4.6). This procedure is unfortunately carried out only in some head and neck units in the UK.

Salivary glands

Experienced surgical excision with facial nerve preservation is the treatment of choice for parotid tumours and submandibular gland lesions. Postoperative radiotherapy may be advisable for high-grade tumours.

Nasal cavity and sinuses

Small tumours are best excised but larger lesions may need maxillectomy or craniofacial resection combined with radiotherapy. Palatal prosthesis offers an alternative to surgical reconstruction.

Neck lumps and lymphomas

Malignant tumours of the neck are usually secondary nodal metastases from a squamous carcinoma of the upper aerodigestive tract or primary lymphomas, although rarely from neuroectodermal tumours. Appropriate investigation will usually reveal the site of an apparently occult primary, which is then treated in combination with the neck as detailed above. Incisional biopsies are best avoided and excision of the neck lump is only carried out:

• if a preliminary FNAC has suggested lymphoma
• if full ENT examination fails to reveal a primary squamous carcinoma site.

If lymphoma is confirmed on histology, further appropriate investigation and treatment are carried out, depending on the type determined by immunocytochemistry. For squamous carcinoma nodes with an occult primary, a neck dissection is performed with postoperative radiotherapy if appropriate and careful follow-up.

Preadmission clinic

After detailed investigation and assessment of the tumour and general medical condition, the patient is seen in the multidisciplinary clinic where the consultant in charge of overall care and his or her colleagues will have discussed and agreed on the course of treatment. At the subsequent preadmission clinic all aspects of treatment and care are checked with the patient and family so that they are fully informed. Sympathetic repetition of many aspects of care will be necessary because the patient will find it difficult to concentrate or take in all details through shock and anxiety after the disturbing diagnosis of cancer.

Physical aspects of treatment can be reinforced, and more readily understood with the use of diagrams, illustrations, anatomical models and equipment. The patient will be able to visualize the normal, and then the altered and reconstructed, anatomical changes in a more logical and sequential way.

Those patients having major head and neck reconstructive surgery or who have an underlying medical problem will be examined and reviewed by the anaesthetist and medical staff, so that any outstanding tests or investigations that have not already been carried out will be completed. The patient and family will also meet any other relevant members of the team to discuss specific aspects of care. The aim of the preadmission clinic is for the patient and family to feel that the whole team is working together for the patient's physical, psychological and social well-being and optimum quality of life, and to facilitate the smooth transition back into society.

Nutrition

The dietitian will assess the patient's nutritional status, and may advise early nutritional support, particularly if the patient has had a prolonged period of dysphagia with weight loss or is otherwise poorly nourished. A nasogastric tube or percutaneous gastrostomy may be required before the start of definitive treatment.

Oral care

Good oral hygiene is essential, particularly if radiotherapy is anticipated as part of the treatment. The dentist and dental hygienist will assess and treat any dental or periodontal disease. Extractions can be planned to be carried out at the time of major surgery rather than put the patient through a second operation. A maxillofacial prosthodontist may also be needed to take any intraoral or facial impressions.

Speech and language therapy

The speech and language therapist will meet any patient who has or may have any speech or hearing impairment. It is vital that they see the speech and language therapist while they are still able to communicate freely in order for them to get to know each other, make assessments and discuss the rehabilitation programme.

Social worker

The social worker can meet the patient, make an assessment, and advise and help with any necessary documentation and employment benefits.

Physiotherapy

Where sacrifice of the accessory nerve at neck dissection is anticipated, a postoperative exercise programme to decrease the degree of shoulder drop and limitation of movement can be discussed.

Clinical nurse specialist

The clinical nurse specialist (CNS) should also meet the patient and family to discuss the rationale for postoperative nursing interventions and the equipment used. This would be at the depth and pace that the patient demanded and would also be supported with illustrations, models, patient booklets and other written materials. The patient may want to tour the head and neck unit or ward at this stage and see where he or she would be nursed. The CNS could also offer advice on any psychological or clinical problems.

Caring for the head and neck cancer patient as part of the multidisciplinary team (see Table 4.1) is one of the most challenging and rewarding areas for nurses. Ideally the core members of the team should meet the patient and family before treatment so that the needs of the patient can be assessed, and advice and reassurance can be given about the anticipated course of treatment and rehabilitation to help allay any fear and anxiety (Rhys Evans, 1996a).

Nursing interventions

Airway management

Airway management and tracheostomy maintenance are two of the most demanding and anxiety-provoking aspects of any nursing care. This mostly stems from fear of potentially acute and life-threatening situations in the head and neck patient because much of the complex surgery involves the common air and food passages. Loss of an adequate airway will lead to death or severe cerebral damage within a few minutes; for this reason it is imperative that nurses caring for this group of patients have a thorough clinical and theoretical knowledge of airway management.

Stridor

Those patients who are temporarily stridulous or who have a compromised airway, not necessitating a tracheostomy, can gain respiratory relief from humidified oxygen or from Heliox (helium and oxygen). Heliox is an extremely valuable gas because the helium gas particles or atoms are smaller than those in normal air and therefore produce less airway resistance if there is a potential obstruction, so that the patient can be ventilated more easily for a temporary period of time.

Tracheostomy care

A tracheostomy can be performed either as a permanent end-tracheostomy procedure such as in a laryngectomy or as a permanent or, more probably, temporary procedure to provide and maintain a patient's airway. In the latter situation obstructions such as tumour or oedema caused by surgery or radiotherapy can be bypassed. A tracheostomy can also be performed to enable the removal of tracheobronchial secretions when the patient is too weak to expectorate independently. Many patients with head and neck cancer also have chronic obstructive airway disease or chronic bronchitis, and may benefit from a tracheostomy to assist in reducing dead space and removal of secretions.

It is essential that a patient who has a tracheostomy should always have, at their bedside or easily accessible, the items mentioned in Table 4.5.

Table 4.5 Essentials for tracheostomy care

1. Humidified oxygen with tracheostomy mask
2. Suction unit with a selection of suction catheters
3. Bowl for water and sodium bicarbonate to clear suction tubing of secretions after suctioning
4. Clean disposable gloves; sterile gloves
5. Two cuffed tracheostomy tubes, one the same size as worn by the patient, the other a size smaller in the event of an emergency tracheostomy tube change
6. One 10-ml syringe to inflate the cuff on the tracheostomy tube
7. A tube of lubricating jelly to facilitate tube insertion
8. Tracheal dilators, in the situation where the tracheostomy tube falls out or where it has been removed and insertion of another tube is difficult. The tracheal dilators can be used to keep the stoma patent until medical assistance arrives (Rhys Evans, 1996a)

Expectoration

The airway should be kept free of secretions at all times and this is most effectively accomplished by encouraging the patient to cough. Not only is the airway cleared, but also the lungs expand to prevent atelectasis and pneumonia.

Suctioning

With a newly formed tracheostomy or if the patient is too weak to cough, the secretions must be suctioned from the trachea as frequently as necessary to keep the airway clear. Deaths from airway obstruction are most commonly the result of inadequate or inexperienced clearing of secretions from the tracheostomy tube or trachea, which may gradually build up over a period of a few hours. This may become critical, particularly at night when the secretions may become more solid with crust formation, eventually causing obstruction.

Suctioning is a clean procedure and sterilized equipment must be used. The catheter should not be inserted further than the carina, and suction should be applied only on withdrawal of the catheter in a gentle rotating movement. The whole procedure should not take longer than 10 seconds but, on completion of the task, the nurse should be absolutely certain that the airway is totally clear and that there is no audible or visible evidence of obstruction.

Fibreoptic tracheoscopy

If there is any doubt about complete clearance of the airway, an appropriate ENT surgeon should be alerted so that he can inspect the tube and trachea with a fibreoptic endoscope, and clear any remaining secretions or crusts.

Type of tube

Various types of tracheostomy tube are available, but for safety it is essential to use one that has a separate inner tube and that is comfortable for the patient. These are available in cuffed, non-cuffed, fenestrated and non-fenestrated forms in different sizes, the use of each of them being indicated for different clinical situations.

Montgomery T-tubes

These tubes, shaped like a 'T', consist of a long vertical Silastic tube which lies in the trachea extending up into the subglottis, with an additional horizontal tube that projects forward through the skin. They may be used after operations for laryngotracheal reconstruction, but can be associated with a problem of crusting at the junction of the horizontal and vertical limbs. The attending nurse must have a clear understanding of the slightly different suctioning and cleaning techniques.

Tube changes

The frequency of tracheostomy tube changes is mostly dependent on the type of secretion. The inner tube may initially have to be changed every half an hour although each patient should be carefully assessed on a continual basis. Any nurse who is starting a span of duty should *always* do a baseline assessment of the airway and tube to check on the type and amount of secretions and the need for humidification or a nebulizing spray.

The outer tube needs changing less frequently but a patient with copious tenacious secretions will need a tube change daily or twice daily, because this is the only way of ensuring that the stoma and tube are free from secretions. It is not uncommon for acute airway obstruction to occur because of a build-up of crusts at the bottom end of a tracheostomy tube that is not recognized unless the whole tube is changed. If patients have minimal secretions, they may need only a weekly tube change.

Laryngectomy tubes or stoma buttons

Some of these do not have an inner tube and will therefore need to be changed frequently, especially when they are first used. Whenever the tube is removed, it is essential that the airway be checked with a torch to ensure that there are no crusts building up below the tube. These can be removed carefully with angled forceps.

Peristomal wounds

Those patients with wounds in or around the stoma (see Figure 4.5) will need to have their tube removed in order to get good visualization of the wound and thorough access for cleaning. Figure 4.5 shows a peristomal infection after a pharyngolaryngectomy with a free jejunum graft. The Foley catheter is placed through the tracheo-oesophageal voice fistula tract during surgery for postoperative feeding. Once oral feeding is established the catheter is removed and replaced with the voice valve (see Figure 4.6).

Tracheostomy dressing

The tracheostomy dressing should be renewed and the circumference of the stoma cleaned and dried at least once, if not twice, a day or more frequently depending on mucus production, to ensure that secretions are cleared and do not lie wet against the skin, causing excoriation. The dressing procedure can be done without removing the tube if appropriate.

Self-care

The patient and family will experience feelings of apprehension and uncertainty over an altered airway. Therefore, it is important that the nursing staff manage and teach the patient and family how to care for the airway in a calm, sensible and logical way. Sharing one's knowledge in this manner will reduce anxiety and build confidence and trust for the patient and family. The main priority is to support and encourage the patient to feel confident in changing the inner tubes of their tracheostomy tube, humidifying with a nebulizing spray, and expectorating secretions independently. Once skilled in these three aspects they will be able to keep the tracheostomy tube patent. It should be remembered that each patient and his or her circumstances are different – some patients feel ready to learn all aspects of care from changing the tracheostomy dressing to doing a complete tube change, whereas others need considerable support.

Laryngectomy

The laryngectomy patient will need to learn all aspects of stomal care and what to do in the event of an emergency. The permanency of the condition makes laryngectomy patients realize that their freedom, independence and survival depend on their knowledge and practical care. However, this type of permanent stoma is easier to manage and laryngectomy tubes are very rarely needed in the long term. Stoma buttons or stoma vents (Rhys Evans, 1996b) are much easier to use but may not be necessary for permanent use.

Wound care

Astute and skilled nursing intervention is necessary for the care of head and neck wounds, which often involve intricate reconstructive techniques. It is essential that specialist head and neck nursing attention is available throughout the wound healing process, to deal with these complex wounds which are at a high risk of developing serious complications.

In the first 24 hours, the patient will be nursed on a one-to-one basis for close observation and monitoring, sometimes in a high-dependency unit, particularly if there is a flap reconstruction. The patient needs to be nursed in a semi-sitting position because gravity will help to reduce oedema. Basic wound observation remains the same but specific observations are necessary for skin flaps.

Skin flaps

A skin flap is composed of skin and subcutaneous tissue and survives provided that it continues to have an intact and functioning arterial and venous circulation. There are two main types of skin flap: free and pedicle.

Free flap

This is obtained from bowel, skin, subcutaneous tissue and sometimes muscle/bone with a main artery and vein, which is separated and then transferred from one area of the body to another. Using microvascular techniques, the artery and vein are anastomosed to a recipient artery and vein in the neck.

Pedicle flap

Skin, subcutaneous tissue, muscle and occasionally bone are transferred from one area to another, but the base or pedicle remains attached to its original blood supply.

The aim of nursing care of any type of flap is to ensure flap viability. Frequent and thorough observation, at least every 15–30 minutes in the immediate postoperative period for the first 24 hours is essential. Circulation is paramount to the flap's survival. Blood flow into the flap must be adequate and blood draining from the flap must also be unobstructed. The skin flap should be pink, warm and blanch, showing brisk capillary return when touched.

Flap monitoring

Various methods have been described and obviously monitoring depends on whether the flap is visible (e.g. in the mouth or neck) or not (hypopharyngeal reconstruction). When pricked the flap should bleed if the circulation is adequate, but if the arterial supply is compromised the flap will become pale and cold and will not bleed. It must be remembered, however, that the normal colour for the flap is the same as its original donor site, which is often paler than mucosal areas within the mouth, although after some months the colour does change (see Figure 4.4). Arterial devascularization is more commonly seen in the first 24 hours after operation. A blue or dusky discoloration indicates venous congestion and this may occur later after several days.

Tapes and dressings

There should be no kinking, tension or pressure on the flap. Vigilant attention must be given to ensure that the tracheostomy tapes, dressing tapes and bandages are not tied too tightly around the flap or wound. Care should also be taken with Hudson or tracheostomy mask tapes to ensure that they are not too tight around the neck, thus impeding blood flow. Oxygen tubing and other lines should not lie over the wound or flap site, causing pressure.

Observation of mottling, duskiness or sudden tightness of the neck dressing can be indicative of haematoma formation and flap or possibly impending flap failure. Bandages used around the neck can also have the disadvantage of preventing visualization of important signs of skin changes, and are generally not needed when suction drainage is used. Fans should be used with caution because they can cause a vasoconstriction of the flap with subsequent failure. The patient should be kept warm to avoid vasoconstriction.

Drainage bottles

All drainage bottles must be patent and checked regularly because a devacuumed or clamped bottle can cause flap failure. If the Redivac tubing is temporarily clamped for movement of the patient, it is essential that it be reopened.

Fluid balance

The patient must have an adequate fluid balance. The haemoglobin should ideally be over 10 grams; if below this the patient should be transfused to ensure that sufficient oxygen is perfusing all wound areas. When a flap is being used, the haemoglobin should not be too high because the blood circulation may become more sluggish, which may jeopardize the circulation particularly in the first few days after operation.

Flap failure

The medical team must be notified immediately if the flap is showing any signs of failure. Flaps can tolerate only about 4 hours of ischaemia before irreversible tissue necrosis occurs. The team will assess the situation and start medical intervention to save the flap if necessary. Such measures may include releasing one or two vital sutures to ease pressure or tension, and evacuating a haematoma, which can be done on the ward or may necessitate the patient going back to the operating theatre.

Free flaps

The flap failure rate should be under 6–10% in experienced units, but a number of flaps may need to be explored if there is any doubt about the circulation. This may be the result of kinking of the pedicle or haematoma formation, but it is essential that a compromised flap be recognized early to allow immediate surgical intervention. Generally for free flaps survival is an 'all-or-nothing' phenomenon because the circulation failure is usually in the main artery or vein. Salvage of a compromised flap is an emergency to evacuate the clot and/or redo the anastomosis because a delay of even an hour may mean that the flap cannot be saved.

Pedicle flaps

The most commonly used flaps in reconstruction of the head and neck are the deltopectoral cutaneous flap and the pectoralis major and latissimus dorsi myocutaneous flaps. These are robust flaps with a good blood supply, although sometimes the distal part of a cutaneous flap may become dusky over a period of a few days and may be lost. Myocutaneous flaps rely on the circulation from perforating vessels of the underlying muscle; if the circulation is poor or compromised because of postoperative oedema, haematoma or a tight overlying skin bridge, the skin surface may become pale, blotchy or congested, depending on whether the venous and/or arterial supply is compromised. For a latissimus dorsi flap, simple abduction and support of the arm may greatly improve the circulation if this is compressed as it goes through the axilla. In general the blood supply to the muscle is good and this usually remains viable even if some of the skin has been lost. For pedicle flaps circulatory changes often happen over a few days and, as any tissue loss is partial, one may adopt a 'wait-and-see' policy if there is no obvious acute cause.

Leeches

Another simple, non-evasive and painless measure to reduce congestion in a flap is by the application of leeches. Each leech can remove/suck approximately 10 ml of blood. Three or four leeches can be applied as necessary in the acute situation to the congested area and may be all that is necessary to ease the tension and improve blood flow. Improvements in the skin colour are noticed almost immediately. With a skilled, professional and empathetic approach, patients will understand and comply, especially as the alternative could be a lengthy surgical procedure.

Early detection combined with prompt expert management can save a flap and prevent putting the patient through further surgery and disfigurement that would occur if a replacement flap had to be harvested.

Skin grafts

Skin grafts are composed of a thin layer of epidermal tissue and a layer of dermis. Skin grafts vary in thickness dependent on the recipient area to be covered. They may be full thickness (Wolfe graft), which is often taken from the postauricular sulcus or the inguinal region, but the most commonly used type of skin graft is split thickness (Thiersh graft), which may be taken from the upper arm or thigh. The skin graft is removed from the donor site and sutured or laid on the recipient area. It acts as a dressing to cover the wound site and eventually becomes incorporated as skin epidermis. A Thiersh graft may also be taken from the buttocks because this is a useful area, especially if the patient is worried about potential scarring and disfigurements at the donor site. Even with the smallest amount of clothing cover, such as bikini bottoms, trunks or underwear, the graft area would be covered.

Nursing observation and care will include both the donor site and the recipient site. The protective covering of the donor site will depend on the surgeon's preference. Commonly tulle gras with cotton wool and a crepe bandage pressure dressing are used. Transparent dressings such as Opsite or an alginate such as Keltostat can also be used (Rhys Evans, 2003). The cotton wool pressure dressing remains *in situ* for about 14 days. Alginate can be removed at an earlier time of 5–7 days.

If the wound leaks excessive exudates, the top dressing can be taken down and re-bandaged. However, if the exudate looks or smells infected the dressing should be soaked off and assessed.

When it is time for the dressing to be removed it should be gently soaked off in the bath or shower. Re-epithelialization occurs in the donor site area as the healing process takes place. For this reason removal of the dressing must never be forced because the granulation tissue will be damaged.

Patients often complain that most of their pain is at the donor site area postoperatively. Some anaesthetists will give a regional nerve block to ease the pain on the donor limb, particularly if it has been bilateral. A local injection of bupivacaine (Marcain) can also dull the pain in the early postoperative period. The pain is the result of exposure of nerve endings. Regular analgesia and avoidance of friction from nightclothes and bedding is essential.

The donor site is often exposed to air while healing occurs. If this is too painful in the early days, a non-adherent dressing such as mepital or Geliperm can be used. It is essential that the area is reassessed every day, with a view to exposing it to the air to dry as soon as the patient can tolerate this. If it is covered for too long, the area becomes wet and infected. Once the area has begun to dry, moisturizing cream can be applied to prevent crust formation and to ease any discomfort. The massaging effects of the cream are very beneficial in preventing taut scar tissue and facilitating formation of a smooth supple skin. Fragrance-free homoeopathic creams are ideal, such as calendula or aloe vera, but any non-perfumed cream will suffice. Arnica cream is helpful to ease discomfort where there is excessive bruising and can be used as long as the skin is intact (Rhys Evans, 2002).

Wound complications

A wound complication is not only distressing and discouraging for the patient and medical staff, but it also invariably means a prolonged stay in hospital.

Fistulas

Fistulas occur quite commonly after major resections of the oral cavity and pharynx, and happen more frequently after 'salvage' surgery because of the damaging effects of radiotherapy on potential healing. Management requires patience and perseverance, and smaller fistulas will gradually close spontaneously although the larger fistulas may need surgical intervention. Keeping the fistula clean, free from infection and as dry as possible may at times be very demanding but will encourage healing (see Figures 4.5 and 4.6).

Sloughing wounds

Sloughing wounds require surgical débridement and/or the use of a topical desloughing agent.

Fungating and malodorous wounds

Fungating and malodorous wounds can be covered with carbon-impregnated dressings and topical antibiotics can be applied such as metronidazole, which is an excellent deodorizer. Metronidazole taken systemically is also most effective for malodorous wounds.

Vascular wounds

Vascular wounds can be dressed with alginate products such as Keltostat.

Intraoral bleeding

Intraoral bleeding can be controlled by rinsing with tranexamic acid.

Major arterial bleeds

Major arterial bleeds can be potentially fatal for some patients but even more minor ones can be very distressing. A massive haemorrhage is usually heralded over the preceding hours by more minor episodes of bleeding, and the source of any minor bleeding must be investigated very carefully. Patients with a previous history of irradiation and who have had a fistula or infection are most at risk if the wound has broken down. The patient should be cannulated and intravenous diamorphine or midazolam (Hypnovel) prescribed in the event of a major arterial haemorrhage. The cannula is also an access route for emergency blood products if the patient needs resuscitation. In the event of a major bleed, the nurse must wear gloves, apply firm pressure with large pads and call for emergency assistance. The rest of the team can administer artificial resuscitation and coordinate operating theatre staff if appropriate (Rhys Evans, 1996b).

Pain management

Between 40% and 80% of patients suffering from head and neck cancer experience pain in various forms at different phases as a result of the disease and/or its treatment. It is often difficult to assess and not always easy to elicit the exact cause because of the complex structure of the head and neck and its diverse sensory innervation. It is imperative to have available a medical specialist in pain management, who has a good understanding of head and neck disease and treatment, to help control this symptom (Bonica, 1985).

Access for administration of analgesia is an important issue for the head and neck patient because swallowing is often difficult or inadvisable during the early postoperative phase. The gastrointestinal tract is almost always functional and therefore a nasogastric tube or gastrostomy is the preferred option for delivery, except during the first 24 hours or so when intravenous opiates may be required. Aspirin-based products should be stopped 10-14 days preoperatively and after surgery they should be used with great caution because they interfere with haemostasis and may predispose to postoperative haematoma formation (Rhys Evans, 1996b).

Complementary methods are also of value in pain management in addition to prescribed regular analgesic medication. Such techniques include acupuncture, diversional therapy, massage and aromatherapy. Constant monitoring of the effectiveness of the pain management regimen should be continued throughout the patient's course of treatment and at follow-up appointments.

Mouth care

Most patients with cancer of the upper gastrointestinal tract, particularly of the mouth and pharynx, will experience problems with mouth care (Table 4.6). This may be caused by the tumour itself, which might interfere with saliva production, lip seal or swallowing, and there is almost always secondary infection and often bleeding. Mouth care problems may also arise as a result of treatment whether surgery, radiotherapy or chemotherapy, or due to an enforced change of diet.

Table 4.6 Mouth care problems in the head and neck cancer patient

Tumour-related problems	Treatment-related problems	
Bleeding	Radiotherapy	
Ulceration	Immediate	– mucositis, ulceration
Pain	Intermediate	– loss of taste (2–3 months)
Infection	Long term:	– loss of saliva
Loose teeth		– dental infection, gingivitis
Inability to swallow		– radionecrosis – mucosal
		– mandibular
	Surgery	
	Early:	– loss of swallowing function
		– flap monitoring and viability
		– oedema, pain, bleeding
		– trismus, loss of lip seal
		– infection, fistulas
	Long term:	– loss of sensation
		– altered muscle function
	Chemotherapy	– ulceration, mucositis
	General	– change of diet

The aim of comprehensive mouth care is to maintain good oral hygiene, to prevent plaque build-up, dental decay and infection, and to minimize pain. It is also essential to keep the oral mucosa moist and intact and to promote patient comfort and well-being. To help achieve good oral status, the patient must be adequately hydrated and the appropriate instruments, solutions and methods used.

Incapacitated patients and those unable to perform their own oral toilet are most at risk from developing mouth problems. It is essential that the nurse makes a thorough assessment of the patient's oral status and assists him or her in arranging the most appropriate regimen.

Irrigation of the oral cavity is very beneficial when the patient has an intraoral lesion or surgical site and helps to keep the mouth or any cavities fresh and clean. It stimulates blood supply, reduces oedema, helps to alleviate pain and discomfort, controls odour, and helps to prevent and clear debris and infection. Irrigation is particularly important when there is altered or reduced sensation (e.g. free flap reconstruction of the tongue or floor of mouth) or when tongue mobility has been affected. When the patient is learning to irrigate, the nurse assists by offering support and advice as well as guidance in order to avoid trauma to exposed tissues, flaps or grafts.

If the oral cleaning is painful or uncomfortable, the patient must be offered analgesia half an hour before the oral hygiene regimen. There will be periods when the patient feels overwhelmed by the many additional aspects of care and rehabilitation that he or she is trying to manage, such as tracheostomy care and enteral feeding. It is therefore both practical and sensible to keep all of these regimens as simple and as logical as possible for optimum patient compliance, especially if they are going to be long term (Rhys Evans, 1996b).

Communication

One of the most difficult problems facing a large proportion of patients with cancer of the aerodigestive tract, particularly during the early postoperative period, is loss of the vital function of communication. This may be temporary as a result of a tracheostomy; there may be laryngeal or tongue oedema from radiotherapy or from the effects of the tumour, or there may be

severe stomatitis. Speech will also be affected after laryngectomy, glossectomy and other oral and pharyngeal reconstruc-
tions for varying periods of time.

The nurse may help by asking questions in such a way that a
yes or no or nod of the head would suffice in the initial postoperative period. Written communication is always made available
such as pen and paper or a magic slate. It should be remembered, however, that nothing irritates a patient more than if the
rushed nurse, doctor or frustrated family member finishes the
patient's sentence for them in their desire to be helpful, particularly if it has been interpreted incorrectly. Family and friends
should be reassured and educated on these points.

Flash cards depicting areas of care are also useful as a temporary measure or for the illiterate patient, as well as appropriate
cards with important words in different languages. Attempting
to communicate will be extremely frustrating at times for
patients, especially if they are feeling depressed or unwell, and it
is vital that the nurse is gentle, encouraging and patient so that
they do not regress or develop complications because of inability to explain symptoms.

Often conversation has to be repeated several times before it
is understood but practice at communication must be encouraged in a safe and private environment. This is particularly
important in the early postoperative period for patients who
have had reconstructive surgery to the mouth or throat when
they might be initially upset at the sound of their altered voice.

Tracheostomy tubes should be fitted with speaking valves as
soon as possible to help ease feelings of isolation for the patient
and facilitate practice of speech. Laryngectomy patients may
have had a tracheo-oesophageal puncture performed either as a
primary or secondary procedure. They will have a Foley
catheter (see Figure 4.5) in the puncture site until they are ready
to be fitted with the surgical voice prosthesis (see Figure 4.6). If
this is done primarily at the time of laryngectomy, the valve is
usually fitted after normal swallowing has been started 7–10
days later. As a secondary procedure the valve can usually be
fitted within 2–3 days (Rhys Evans, 2003).

Psychological support

When a patient is first diagnosed as having cancer, a potentially
life-threatening disease, the initial shock, anger, sense of loss,

lack of control and grief are virtually the same feelings one experiences after bereavement. It is therefore important to recognize that the patient will be in need of the appropriate support. They are grieving the loss of part of themselves and their life as they once knew it, which will never be quite the same again. This sense of loss is much more apparent in cancers of the head and neck because it is so often combined with an important functional disability such as loss of ability to speak or eat normally or with some noticeable facial scarring or flap reconstruction, affecting the patient's fundamental 'persona'.

If the patient's symptoms are controlled or minimal, it is hoped that a relatively normal lifestyle can be resumed including returning to work, even after total laryngectomy, with a near-normal voice. Various studies have found that patients who maintain close relationships with their family and friends are more likely to cope with the course of their treatment and rehabilitation (Wortman and Dunkel-Schetter, 1979).

Patients will experience a degree of depression at some stage in their illness and this too must be recognized as a normal response to the threat of disfigurement, dysfunction and possibly death. The patient and family must be given the opportunity, time and privacy to express their anxiety and fears.

Once the period of grieving has begun, the diagnosis of cancer can also precipitate the onset of the patient's coping mechanisms, as recognized by Caplan in 1966. Most patients demonstrate an extraordinarily brave determination to get on with their life, whatever their dysfunction and/or disfigurement, especially if the alternative is death (Rhys Evans, 1993). The majority of patients employ a coping mechanism that we all practise to some extent in our lives – that of social comparison. They frequently compare themselves with others, with the subconscious intent to be in a stronger, more positive position. By comparing their handicaps with those of others, they will reason that to lose their ear or voice or part of their tongue, for example, is better than to lose an eye or to be confined to a wheelchair for life. By making these comparisons, patients try to relieve some of their fate and enhance the value and quality of their life.

Helping patients and their families to express themselves, and feel comfortable to interact with the staff involved with their care, will foster trust and reassurance, with the knowledge that everyone is seen to be working together to achieve an acceptable quality of life. Some patients and families may want to talk to someone who is not involved in their immediate care. Often referral to a mental health professional or support group can be helpful.

Sexual health

Sexual health must be addressed if the head and neck cancer patients' care is to be covered in its entirety. Whether in health or sickness, we are all sexual beings with the fundamental needs of being loved and desired, and of finding comfort in another person.

Sexual expression

The need to support sexual expression in patients with cancer, or any illness for that matter, confirms their vitality, and being able to talk about it gives confidence in their survival (Rhys Evans, 1996b). It may not be appropriate to discuss sexual health problems with all patients. One may not feel comfortable in doing so, but in these cases it does not mean that the situation should be overlooked. The patient should be referred to someone who is more comfortable and qualified in discussing sexual health issues such as the CNS or another member of the head and neck team (Rhys Evans, 2003).

When is the best time to talk about sexual health issues? The patient needs to know that they have permission to broach the subject and that it will not be a matter of shock or embarrassment. Preoperatively, a gentle way of initiating the subject of appearance and attractiveness may be when the operative procedure is discussed, e.g. if the patient is going to have a split-skin graft taken and they have a choice of where the donor site can be, the patient can be asked for his or her preference. It can be suggested that some people like to wear shorts or sleeveless shirts if they feel they have nice legs or attractive arms. Does the patient have a personal preference? The skin can alternatively be taken from the buttocks so that the area would be covered in most situations (Rhys Evans, 2003).

If the patient is to have a myocutaneous flap, in a female the latissimus dorsi flap is cosmetically much more acceptable than a pectoralis major flap. It might be possible to make the incision in a more horizontal fashion so that the scar can be covered by a bra or bikini top. By adopting this approach, the patient will recognize that it is accepted as normal that they will be concerned about their appearance. We all have aspects of our body that we prefer and it is important that the patient recognizes that the head and neck surgical team is aware of these potential sources of concern, and that they will take these personal factors into consideration.

Oral expression

Many head and neck surgical procedures involve breaching the integrity of the oral cavity. Research has shown that sexual adjustment is a common concern for the patient, especially if the mouth is affected, because this plays an important role in oral stimulation and expression (Rhys Evans, 1993). Most patients complain that they cannot enjoy a proper kiss or cuddle with their partner or kiss their children properly, and long for the warmth, intimacy and reassurance that this provides.

Facial expression

Limitations in spontaneous facial expressions are also frustrating and inhibiting for sexual expression, and these concerns should be addressed if there is likely to be potential weakness of the facial nerve or facial muscles.

Sputum

Sputum production, particularly if copious from the oral cavity or uncontrollable from a stoma, is another major concern. Patients worry that they appear dirty as well as unattractive. Agents that help dry up the secretions can be a useful temporary measure. For stoma patients, in the early days of their sexual rehabilitation or until their confidence increases with their new stoma, practical suggestions can be made such as filling a bathroom with steam from the bath or shower, which will in turn humidify the patient's stoma (Rhys Evans, 2002). Bathing together can be incorporated as foreplay with their partner. Alternative positions for lovemaking can also be suggested if the patient is anxious about coughing over his or her partner.

With sensitivity, ingenuity and appropriate humour, most patients' anxiety can be relieved. It is imperative, however, that the patient and family feel reassured of complete trust and confidentiality (Rhys Evans, 2003).

Cosmetic camouflage

A cosmetic camouflage service and a good prosthetics department are also vital for some patients in helping them to regain their identity and confidence in facing their partner, family and the public.

Continuing support

Information on support services and groups must be made available for those patients who would like to attend. It is important to continue to enquire in the follow-up clinics how the patient is coping at home and if they have any relationship or personal worries, because many problems sometimes manifest only when the patient is back at home. It may be appropriate for the patient to be followed up in the CNS-led clinic (or equivalent clinic) for ongoing psychological, social or sexual health support, which also ensures continuity for the patient. In the general follow-up clinic where the patient may meet a new or different member of the medical team, it is often difficult or inappropriate to discuss personal matters. Patients are usually concerned only with one vital medical issue – that they are still free of cancer.

Palliative care

Cancer of the upper aerodigestive tract is mainly a locoregional disease and only a small proportion die from distant metastases. Progressive uncontrolled tumours in the head and neck present some of the most distressing problems for a patient, relatives and carers (Table 4.7).

Table 4.7 Potential terminal problems in head and neck cancer

Problems	Suggested solutions
Severe pain	Opiate analgesia ± adjuvant medication
Airway obstruction	May require tracheostomy
Progressive dysphagia	Relieved by PEG or nasogastric tube
Loss of voice	Involvement of the larynx or oral cavity
Infected fungating tumour Leaking fistulas	Vigilant wound care and mouth care
Gross oedema of the tongue, face and neck from lymphatic obstruction	Symptomatic relief, keep area cool, gentle massage to aid lymphatic flow
Carotid bleed	Reassurance

PEG, percutaneous endoscopic gastrostomy.

These distressing and disfiguring problems may also inevitably cause intense psychological disturbance from loss of communication, change in body image, loss of self-esteem and attractiveness, particularly to children or grandchildren who do not fully comprehend. Great skill, experience and empathy are essential in helping these unfortunate patients during their last few weeks or months to die with dignity and minimal distress.

Conclusion

For the patient with cancer of the upper aerodigestive tract, optimum effective management requires intensive, comprehensive nursing and a unified holistic approach to care with the medical staff and multidisciplinary team from the very outset. Thoughtful preparation preoperatively and assiduous skilled nursing after surgery will offer the patient optimum opportunity to regain, in their perception, a quality of life that is acceptable after the impact of head and neck cancer and its treatment. The delivery of this care should be with total empathy and consideration at all times.

References

Bonica JJ (1985) Treatment of cancer pain: current status and future needs. In: Fields HL (ed.), Advances in Pain and Therapy, Vol 9. New York: Raven Press, pp. 589–617.

Caplan G (1996) Principles of Preventative Psychiatry. London: Basic Books

Rhys Evans F (1993) An investigation into functional problems following major oral surgery in head and neck cancer patients, and coping mechanisms employed by the patient. MSc Thesis, University of Surrey.

Rhys Evans F (1996a) Tracheostomy care and laryngectomy voice rehabilitation. In: Mallett J, Bailey C (eds), The Royal Marsden NHS Trust, Manual of Clinical Nursing Procedures. London: Blackwell Science, pp. 550–565.

Rhys Evans F (1996b) Tumours of the head and neck. In: Tschudin V (ed.), Nursing the Patient with Cancer. London: Prentice Hall, pp. 178–201.

Rhys Evans F (2003) Nursing care of the head and neck cancer patient. In: Rhys Evans PH, Gullane P, Montgomery P, Gluckman J (eds), Tumours of the Head and Neck. London: Isis, in press.

Rhys Evans PH, Henk JM (2003) Incidence, aetiology and multidisciplinary management of head and neck cancer. In: Rhys Evans PH, Gullane P, Montgomery P, Gluckman J (eds), Tumours of the Head and Neck. London: Isis, in press.

Robin PE et al. (1983) Incidence and survival of head and neck cancer. In: Rhys Evans PH, Fielding J, Robin PE (eds), Head and Neck Cancer. London: Wiley: Liss.

Wortman CB, Dunkel-Schetter C (1979) Interpersonal relationships and cancer: A theoretical analysis. Journal of Clinical Issues 39: 120–155.

CHAPTER 5

Cancer of the upper gastrointestinal tract

KAREN TARHUNI, HANIF SHIWANI AND PETER SEDMAN

The nurse practitioner (NP) in upper gastrointestinal (GI) care has a highly specialized role and works as a pivotal member of a multidisciplinary team to maintain and improve standards of care while developing nursing practice that is supported by scientific evidence. The NP will be involved in the assessment, management and ongoing support of patients with GI and hepatobiliary disease. The role involves the following:

- Preparation of patients undergoing investigation of serious GI pathology which will include emotional and psychological support.
- Patient educator relating to the diagnosis and treatment options for pathologies uncovered.
- Continuous in-hospital and community support for patients and their families.
- Undertaking gastroscopy for diagnosis after GI symptoms, placing gastrostomy tubes and provision of support after placement of oesophageal stent.
- Acting as a resource and educator for other healthcare professionals.
- Ensuring that practice meets evidence-based guidelines and coordinating clinical audit and research.

This chapter outlines some of the causes and treatments associated with cancer of the upper GI tract. Surgical options and medical treatments are considered, although it is important to recognize that health care based on evidence is constantly evolving.

Assessment

The potential benefits of assessment by the NP include:

- Patients and their relatives are prepared for admission and discharge by involvement of the NP at an early stage, helping to allay fear and anxiety normally associated with hospital procedures and serious pathology (Wilson-Barnett and Carrigy, 1978; Gordon, 1987).
- Efficient use of hospital beds/operating theatre time.
- Decreased cancellation rates on the day of surgery as a result of inadequate patient preparation and selection.

An effective assessment is the basis from which support and instruction can be individualized for each patient. Patients must be provided with information relating to their disease or condition, presented in a way best suited to meet each patient's motor ability and sensory needs. During assessment, the NP should systematically assimilate and communicate information in order to understand each patient's physical and mental state, along with related experiences and expectations.

The assessment process should be used to support diagnosis and facilitate admission requirements. A structured format can be employed to define a recognized model of care, which in turn can support data collection, e.g. Gordon (1987) suggests that the following may be incorporated:

- Health perception and health management, assessment of the patient's perceived pattern of health, well-being and management of health.
- Nutritional and metabolic status, including consumption of food and fluids.
- Elimination, looking at patterns of excretion.
- Cognitive–perceptual level, examining sensory and psychological status.
- Sleep and rest cycles, ascertaining patterns of sleep, rest and relaxation.
- Self-perception, considering the individual's feelings of body image and comfort.
- Interpersonal issues, examining relationships and engagements.
- Sexuality, observing for difficulties or dissatisfaction.

- Coping, generally looking for effectiveness in terms of stress tolerance.
- Value beliefs, considering spiritual and personal goals that guide choices and decisions.

Using this model Gordon (1987) focuses the assessment to determine the patient's level of function within each category. Much of the history should be organized around the factors affecting ingestion and elimination, determining the presence and extent of upper GI alterations, with the assessment supported by physical examination and diagnostic test results. Biographical information, such as history of presenting symptoms, past medical history and family medical history, is also a very important part of the initial assessment process. Obviously, future assessments will not need to be as extensive; merely updating the patient's symptoms should be sufficient.

Symptoms of upper GI disease

The symptoms commonly experienced by people with upper GI cancers include dysphagia (difficulty in swallowing or the sensation of food sticking), dyspepsia (pain or discomfort soon after eating) and upper abdominal pain. Weight loss is another important symptom and many will experience nutritional deficiencies as a result of nausea, vomiting, early satiety or a range of swallowing difficulties. The finding of anaemia should alert one to the possibility of an upper GI cancer and investigations of both the upper and lower GI tract should be considered in the newly diagnosed anaemic patient, particularly when the patient is elderly and where no other obvious cause is apparent.

Investigations of upper GI disease

The general principle of investigation is to assess the clinical suspicions and obtain objective evidence of any tissue damage. Following on from that, investigations to stage the tumour and to determine the status of local and distant metastases should be performed. The immediate aim of surgical intervention is to alleviate symptoms and to improve quality of life, with the long-term aim being to improve survival.

Endoscopy

Upper GI endoscopy (UGIE), also known as oesophagogastro-duodenoscopy (OGD) or gastroscopy, allows visualization of the mucosa of the oesophagus, stomach and duodenum, assessing for tumours, vascular changes, mucosal inflammation, ulcers, hernias or obstruction. In addition to these diagnostic functions, the gastroscope enables tissue specimens for biopsy to be taken, polyps to be removed or active bleeding sources to be coagulated or banded. It may also be used to facilitate dilatation of strictures and placement of stents or gastrostomy tubes. It is perhaps the most common investigative test for upper GI symptoms and is usually performed as an outpatient procedure either under sedation or by using a local anaesthetic throat spray.

Gastroscopy is the mainstay of the investigation and diagnosis of oesophageal and gastric cancers, and is widely employed to detect these tumours at as early a stage as is possible.

A variant of this test is endoscopic retrograde cholangiopancreatography (ERCP), which allows assessment and treatment of bile duct problems.

Ultrasonography

Ultrasonography is a non-invasive test involving assessment of the patterns of reflections of echoes sent back from internal organs when ultrasound waves are passed through them. It is especially useful in looking at solid internal organs, stones or fluid collections in the abdomen, but is less effective in looking at organs deep to gas-filled bowel because the gas distorts the images too much.

Computed tomography

This is a sophisticated radiological procedure involving X-rays and powerful computers, which allow the construction of detailed images of the soft and bony tissues in any selected transverse (axial) plane of the body. This procedure helps the identification and staging of upper GI pathology, especially tumours and lymph node enlargements, and is very useful in assessing the site and cause of intestinal obstructions.

Barium swallow and meal

Although largely replaced by endoscopy, this investigation is still very useful in specific situations or to complement circumstances where endoscopy is equivocal. The patient swallows barium and as he or she does so radiographs are taken to monitor the progress of the barium. In the oesophagus, the passage of barium is assessed by video radiograph (video barium swallow) whereas in the stomach standard radiographs are taken at timed intervals (barium meal) to look for subtle anatomical changes or to assess extramucosal disease.

Blood tests

Haemoglobin

Anaemia is common in patients with GI malignancy and malnutrition. This is most commonly the result of chronic slow bleeding from a tumour or ulcer, but may also be secondary to absorptive problems (vitamin B_{12} absorption in pernicious anaemia or iron absorption in coeliac disease).

Total lymphocyte count

This reflects immunological competence and may reflect poor nutritional status. Although levels may be depleted with malignancy, they are also reduced in zinc deficiency and non-specific stress.

Plasma proteins

Many patients presenting with upper GI disease may have poor and deteriorating nutritional status. Low levels of plasma protein may be a reflection of this. The long half-life of albumin (20 days) makes it an insensitive marker of nutritional status; however, prealbumin and retinal-binding protein have much shorter half-lives (2 days and 10 hours, respectively) and therefore they are more sensitive indicators of nutritional depletion. The transferrin level may also give an indication of protein calorie status.

Oesophageal cancer

Worldwide, carcinoma of the oesophagus is the ninth most common cancer, of which 80% of new cases occur in developing countries (Parkin et al., 1993). The highest incidences reported occur in localized areas of Japan, China and Brazil

(Muir et al., 1987). In the UK, oesophageal cancer comprises about 5% of all carcinomas and causes about 4000 deaths each year. The reported male:female ratio of oesophageal cancer is 2:1, with most cases occurring in the over-60 age group.

Histologically oesophageal cancer may be divided into two primary histological subtypes: squamous cell carcinoma and adenocarcinoma. Squamous cell carcinomas are, overall, the more common type of tumour and this type of cancer may be seen throughout the length of the gullet. The slightly less common subtype is adenocarcinoma, which is derived from glandular cells and tends to occur in the lower oesophagus. Some (5%) are true adenocarcinomas of the oesophagus, arising within columnar cells of the oesophagus and may be at any level, but most are of gastric type origin spreading upwards, some occurring within hiatus hernias.

In recent years there has been a dramatic increase in the incidence of this latter subtype of oesophageal adenocarcinoma for reasons that are incompletely understood.

There is a strong association between oesophageal cancers and the environment, with a strong interrelationship of squamous cell carcinoma, alcohol and tobacco. Gastro-oesophageal reflux disease (GORD) and oesophagitis have been linked to adenocarcinoma of the oesophagus. Chronic oesophagitis may also be recognized as a predisposing condition, which in the context of Barrett's oesophageal change is characterized by polypoid or flat mucosa.

Macroscopically three subtypes of oesophageal cancer can be recognized:

- annular stenosing lesion usually found at the lower oesophagus/gastric cardia
- epitheliomatous ulcer with raised everted edges
- fungating cauliflower-like friable mass.

Predisposing factors for oesophageal cancer have been identified and include achalasia, chemical strictures, tylosis, Plummer–Vinson/Patterson–Brown–Kelly syndrome, oesophageal diverticulae and previous chest irradiation. Perhaps the most important is the appearance of Barrett's oesophagus. This is defined as the replacement of the squamous epithelium (designed to withstand physical trauma) by a columnar-lined adenomatous mucosa in the lower oesophagus – a cellular change that is known as metaplasia (Barrett, 1950). Usually this is regarded as a consequence of chronic gastro-oesophageal reflux because adenomatous mucosa is particularly suited to withstand chemical trauma and it is thought that acid or occasionally biliary reflux leads to this cellular change. Metaplastic change may induce a genetic instability in the cells predisposing them to malignant change. The exact sequence of events remains controversial, but it is noted that the risk of developing an adenocarcinoma with Barrett's oesophagus is between 30 and 40 times that of the general population.

Presenting symptoms

By far the most common symptom is the sensation of food sticking in the gullet on a regular basis over the period of a few weeks before presentation. This 'dysphagia' may initially be related to specific solid foods (red meat, toast, potato, etc.). The patient may often indicate the level of obstruction on the breastbone with his or her hand. This symptom may be associated with a recent history of weight loss, which in itself does not necessarily imply advanced disease.

Less commonly, tumours may be picked up during investigations for a new onset of heartburn in the more elderly patient or of more non-specific indigestion symptoms. Occasionally they may be seen in surveillance endoscopy for Barrett's oesophagus or in the follow-up of dysplastic lesions previously noted on endoscopy. It is uncommon for these tumours to present with bleeding or anaemia. Often the symptoms are late in presenting, hence the difficulty in picking these cancers up at an early stage when treatment has the best chance of success.

Investigations

Oesophagoscopy

This is the primary investigation for the patient with dysphagia and is mandatory. When the dysphagia is very high (at the level of the neck), a contrast swallow is occasionally considered first but this is relatively uncommon.

The endoscopic appearance of oesophageal cancers is frequently very typical, with craggy ulcerating hard lesions or polypoidal lesions, although the diagnosis should always be confirmed by biopsy and histopathology. Sampling errors are not uncommon and, if a tumour is suspected at endoscopy but the biopsy is negative, the endoscopy must be repeated. If necessary, exfoliative cytology (endoscopic brushings of the lesion) may be performed as well.

The appearance of very early squamous cell carcinomas may be very subtle with a simple red or pink area only. The most common appearance is that of a superficial erosive cancer, consisting of a slightly depressed lesion with grey erosions in a reddish mucosa or as whitish elevated plaques with slightly depressed reddened areas. If in doubt biopsy with or without cytology is essential,

Radiology

Computed tomography

Once an oesophageal lesion is diagnosed, staging is mandatory to determine the best treatment option and whether there is a possibility of surgery. In most centres contrast enhanced computed tomography (CT) of the thorax and abdomen is the test of choice and should be instituted without delay. Magnetic resonance imaging (MRI) is also sometimes used for this purpose and CT and MRI may be considered equivalent tests. Local availability and expertise in the radiology department will determine best local practice.

Barium swallow is occasionally useful in confirming the diagnosis when endoscopy is difficult or incomplete.

Ultrasonography

In patients with suspected liver metastases abdominal ultrasonography is often helpful and is a better test to evaluate the liver than either CT or routine MRI. It tends to be reserved for those patients where CT or MRI is equivocal in respect of the liver.

Endoluminal ultrasonography

This is a new technique that is not yet universally available, but which is rapidly being seen as invaluable in determining the stage of the tumour and therefore the patient's suitability for surgical treatment. A thin ultrasonic probe is introduced via a flexible endoscope and manipulated into the lumen of the tumour. The ultrasonic pictures produced allow the local spread of the cancer to be assessed, especially the depth of wall invasion (T level) and the likelihood of local lymph node invasion

(N status). Occasionally the presence of distant metastases may be noted (M status). Initial objections to this technique were based on the possibility of perforating the tumour during the test, but the more modern slim-line probes are much safer.

Bronchoscopy

Midoesophageal cancers may occasionally directly invade the trachea or left main bronchus and in doing so become inoperable. Bronchoscopy is useful in identifying such patients and is employed selectively, based on site of tumour, endoscopic appearance or CT.

Blood tests/tumour markers

Routine blood analysis should be performed. Anaemia may be corrected before any treatment and nutritional status may be assessed. There are no useful tumour markers as yet for use with oesophageal cancers.

Treatment

The treatment depends on the staging of the disease and the presenting condition of the patient. Staging is employed first to determine whether the tumour is localized and therefore potentially curable or whether it has spread and therefore only palliative treatments are appropriate.

Staging is based on the TNM (tumour size, lymph node status, metastases) system, which is outlined in Appendix I. This is a universally accepted system for grading tumours and allows comparison of results from centre to centre.

Once the TNM status has been established, this allows the tumour to be assigned into a particular stage ('1' or localized tumour to '4' or advanced tumour). Stage 1 and 2 disease is usually considered for surgery, with stage 4 disease suitable for palliative treatment only. The situation in stage 3 disease is less clear, largely because it is not always possible preoperatively to determine whether the lymph node enlargement is caused by tumour or a benign cause and, under these circumstances, the benefit of doubt is usually given and surgery offered. If, subsequently, it is found that these nodes are involved by tumour the prognosis is often guarded.

Surgery

Surgery is reserved for patients where cure is considered possible. The operations available are all very major procedures with significant risks and should not be considered unless it appears that all of the tumour can be resected in one specimen. It is not appropriate to embark on surgery with a purely palliative intention, because other techniques are preferable in this situation. Surgery involves removal of the tumour, the surrounding lymph nodes, the oesophagus above the tumour and usually also the upper part of the stomach. Although the oesophagus is immobile the stomach is fortunately very mobile and can be moved into the thorax or neck to restore intestinal continuity. The upper stomach is joined to the remaining oesophagus and healing of this join is required before the patient is allowed to eat and drink. Failure of the anastomosis to heal is a major and recognized complication and associated with significant mortality. Even in 'well-selected' patients, the operative mortality rate is about 5–10% and therefore considerable.

Potentially curable tumours may not be treated by surgery if the patient has other significant operative medical risk factors that would prevent the patient from surviving the operation. As a result of this and because oesophageal cancers tend to present at a late stage, less than 40% of patients are offered surgery even in the most adventurous surgical units.

Four operations are regularly used for oesophagectomy and the choice of these depends on the level of the tumour, the general health of the patient and the surgeon's preference, depending on the hospital in which they work and the support services available to patients pre-, peri- and postoperatively. The important principles associated with surgery are that:

- the tumour be fully excised intact
- as many surrounding lymph nodes as possible are removed
- 10-cm 'clearance' of the oesophagus (or stomach) is achieved above and below the tumour
- the remaining bowel ends are healthy, well vascularized and can be joined together without tension.

The following are the more common operations performed.

Left thoracoabdominal approach

An incision is made in the left chest at the level of the sixth rib, which can be extended along the rib cage into the left upper abdomen. The arch of the aorta may limit access to the midoesophagus in some patients, but otherwise access to the whole oesophagus is possible through one incision.

Ivor Lewis 'two stage' (Lewis, 1947)

In this procedure an abdominal incision is combined with a separate right thoracotomy to allow access to the stomach and its lymph nodes, and to the oesophagus and thoracic lymph nodes, separately. The two incisions cannot be combined because the liver would prevent this, although the improved access to the abdominal lymph nodes persuades some surgeons to adopt this approach. The anastomosis between the mobilized lower stomach and fixed upper oesophagus is made in the chest.

McKeown 'three stage' (McKeown, 1981)

This is a modification of the Ivor Lewis approach in which a third incision is made in the left side of the neck and the stomach mobilized into the neck, where the anastomosis is fashioned. This allows more oesophagus to be removed, and has the advantage that if the join does leak it is more superficial than a leaking anastomosis in the chest, and therefore easier to manage. However, because of the greater distance that the stomach has to be moved, it is possible that the risk of a leak is greater.

Transhiatal oesophagogastrectomy

This approach is favoured in circumstances where the surgeon does not wish to perform a thoracotomy because this part of the operation is usually the most painful and gives rise to some postoperative problems – especially in less well-equipped units. An incision is made in the abdomen and another in the neck, and the intervening oesophagus is stripped out between these two. There is concern that this approach is less diligent in removing lymph nodes in the chest, which may be most important for thoracic oesophageal tumours, but the generally smoother postoperative course may compensate for this disadvantage especially for tumours at the gastro-oesophageal junction where the lymph nodes are often accessible through the abdominal incision.

The choice of operation will therefore depend on various factors and no one operation has been shown to be better overall than another.

Additional, complementary therapies

Cytotoxic chemotherapy

This is a systemic treatment, which may reduce the tumour bulk. Dramatic responses are occasionally seen with complete radiological regression of the tumour. It may, however, be toxic and therefore careful monitoring is required during treatment. This treatment is not known ever to produce a 'cure', although it may occasionally convert an inoperable tumour to a potentially operable one and may improve local symptoms by improving swallowing. Cisplatin/fluorouracil-based regimens are usually used for both adenocarcinomas and squamous cell carcinomas of the oesophagus.

Radiotherapy

This may be delivered by targeted external beam or locally within the oesophageal lumen itself by placing radioactive probes within the oesophagus endoscopically. This approach is known as (endoluminal) brachytherapy and is useful in the control of local symptoms to improve swallowing.

Combination of therapies

Unfortunately the cure rates from surgery are not high and recurrence of tumour is not uncommon, particularly for the more advanced cancers. Combinations of additional treatments are therefore continuously under investigation, in particular combinations of cytotoxic chemotherapy and surgery, and radiotherapy with chemotherapy. These treatments, together with surgery, may be given immediately postoperatively (adjuvant therapy) or preoperatively (neoadjuvant therapy). Adjuvant therapy is considered if the type of tumour removed is known to have a very high risk of recurrence (based on operative findings or subsequent laboratory tests), but must be instituted within 1 month of surgery to be effective because there is no evidence that therapy later than this time has any effect on the patterns of recurrence.

Neoadjuvant therapy (giving the treatment before surgery) was therefore suggested to try to shrink the cancer before the surgeon operates and give surgery a better chance of cure.

Research into the best options is ongoing but at present the administration of two cycles of chemotherapy (currently fluorouracil and leucovorin) before surgery appears to be the most effective approach and is associated with a 10% improvement in overall survival 2 years postoperatively.

Some current trials are investigating the combination of radiotherapy, chemotherapy and surgery, but as yet there is no evidence that giving three treatments is better than giving two and this method is associated with increased complication rates.

Radiotherapy with chemotherapy is considered in patients not suitable for surgery.

Palliative treatments

Patients with advanced tumours, or those who are unfit for surgery, are treated by non-surgical means. Palliation may be directed to the control of local symptoms or to slow the progression of disease. Such treatments include:

- surgical bypass
- endoluminal stent
- endoluminal laser therapy
- alcohol injection.

Surgical bypass

This is now rarely employed because more modern stents are equally effective and less invasive than open surgery.

Endoluminal stenting

Three different approaches to stenting oesophageal cancers are available to permit restoration of swallowing in the patient with dysphagia:

- The classic Mousseau–Barbin or Celestin tubes were traditionally placed at open surgery when, at the time of surgery, it became apparent that the tumour was inoperable. These are now less frequently used because preoperative staging is much more reliable in screening out patients for whom surgery is not possible.
- The Atkinson tube is a silicone tube that is placed endoscopically.
- Self-expanding metal 'wall' stents are usually radiologically directed metal stents, which may be placed across the

tumour and then dilated, compressing the tumour radially and increasing the lumen. Metal stents are the most modern and generally preferred technique, because they remain patent longer than the plastic and silicone stents and are less prone to obstruction. However, once placed they cannot be removed again and they are considerably more expensive than the other types of stent.

There is a risk of oesophageal perforation with the insertion of an oesophageal stent, which may be as high as 20%. Complications of stenting also include late overgrowth or ingrowth of tumour, gastro-oesophageal reflux, incomplete expansion, bolus obstruction, bleeding and pain.

Laser therapy requires the use of a neodymium:yttrium–aluminium garnet laser (Nd:YAG), which was first reported to be effective in oesophageal cancer palliation in 1982. This form of therapy uses a catheter, which is passed through the instrument channel of the endoscope. Under direct vision, the laser beam is directed at the intraluminal tumour to heat and vaporize the tissue and gradually reopen the lumen, thus producing effective recanalization and good swallowing. Unfortunately, one of the main disadvantages of this procedure is that it has to be repeated at regular intervals and is associated with a risk of perforation.

Prognosis of oesophageal cancer

Cancer of the oesophagus carries a generally poor prognosis. Only 40% of patients are suitable for surgery, with the remainder being offered palliative treatment or occasionally radical radiotherapy/chemotherapy. Even in patients undergoing surgery 25% will achieve only a 2-year survival.

Gastric cancer

Gastric cancer remains a common cause of mortality in the Western World. In the UK, it is the third most common cause of cancer death in men and the fourth most common cause in women. The incidence of stomach cancer appears to be falling in parts of the Western World where, at the same time, the incidence of lower oesophageal cancer is rising; dietary factors may in part be responsible for this. Gastric cancer affects men twice as frequently as women and the risk of developing gastric cancer increases with age, reaching a peak in the sixth decade.

Gastric cancer is more common in people in lower socioeconomic groups, again for reasons that are not understood. As with oesophageal cancer, treatment is most effective in the early stages of the disease and early diagnosis is therefore essential.

There is a strong international variation in the incidence of gastric cancer; it is particularly common in Japan and Chile and relatively less common in Europe and North America. When considering this disease, it is sometimes helpful to differentiate the results and philosophy of reports and to distinguish studies as to whether they were conducted in the Western World or in Japan where the approaches and patterns of disease are different, e.g. in Japan screening for gastric cancer is performed because the disease is so common there. Patients therefore tend to present with much earlier lesions and in general are fitter medically and less obese than their European counterparts, sometimes allowing more aggressive treatments to be performed. The results from treatment are correspondingly better in Japan than in the West for patient factors as well as possibly for surgical factors.

Causation

The causative factors in the development of gastric cancer are unclear but are probably a combination of environmental and, to a lesser extent, genetic factors. Genetics must play a part because 4% of patients have a family history of the disease and the clear evidence of familial trends was most famously observed in the Bonaparte family in which Napoleon, his father, grandfather and four siblings all had the disease.

Patients with hypogammaglobulinaemia, pernicious anaemia and certain blood groups may be predisposed to this condition. It is thought, however, that environmental factors are probably more important for most patients. This is evidenced by the very significant geographical variations in the disease that cannot be explained genetically, the changing incidence in some but not all countries, and the higher incidence seen in patients after previous benign gastric surgery. Agents and chemicals thought to be implicated in the disease include bile in the stomach, smoked fish, cigarette smoking and the presence of *Helicobacter pylori* in the stomach. It is possible that the changing use of drugs for peptic ulcers may also have an indirect role.

Adenomatous gastric polyps are considered premalignant lesions, especially when they are more than 2 cm in diameter, but the more common gastric polyps seen on endoscopy are hyperplastic regenerative polyps that are not considered premalignant. The findings of dysplasia or carcinoma *in situ* are regarded as precancerous.

Presenting symptoms

Indigestion, particularly as a new symptom in elderly people, should alert one to the possible presence of gastric cancer, but it may also be the result of benign gastric ulceration. In either event early endoscopy is advised, especially if there is a history of weight loss, anaemia or vomiting. Medical therapy with H$_2$-receptor antagonist drugs or proton pump inhibitor therapy may relieve the symptoms of gastric cancer discomfort temporarily, in the same way as it relieves peptic ulceration pain; this is not in itself a reassuring observation. Endoscopy and biopsy before starting treatment with these drugs are therefore advised.

Often gastric cancers may present with symptoms of bleeding overtly by vomiting blood (haematemesis), by the passage of partially digested blood rectally (melaena) or with simple iron deficiency anaemia. Again endoscopy will be required to differentiate benign from malignant causes.

Distal gastric cancers may obstruct the gastric outlet and cause vomiting, which is often copious, delayed for several hours after a meal and characterized by an absence of bile in the vomitus. More subtly, by delaying gastric emptying, gastric cancers may present with a history of heartburn or reflux disease.

Dysphagia caused by a proximal lesion or simple weight loss is a rarer presentation while some patients present with the effects of metastatic disease. In the UK, over 70% of patients will have had symptoms for 6 months or more by the time of diagnosis.

Types of gastric cancer

The vast majority of gastric cancers are adenocarcinomas (95%) although lymphomas, sarcomas and carcinoid tumours are occasionally seen. Endoscopically, they may appear as elevated mucosal lesions that are sometimes polypoidal in appearance, but they may appear as 'punched-out' ulcers with or without elevated margin. Early gastric cancers may appear as a simple red spot or erythematous patch, and a rare but lethal form of the disease, linitis plastica, presents with no mucosal lesion at all but may be detected by the astute endoscopist as a non-distensible gastric wall on endoscopy. This latter form of the disease is characterized by extensive submucosal spread of the disease and is colloquially called the 'leather bottle' stomach. Sadly, it is rarely detected at a stage where treatment might be possible.

Treatment

Unlike in oesophageal cancer, chemotherapy and radiotherapy have a very limited role because these treatments have yet to be proved effective against stomach cancer progression. Surgery is therefore the mainstay of treatment and is performed once the tumour has been diagnosed and staged. The only delays in planning surgery should be in response to the very occasional need to optimize nutritional status before surgery or to optimize the patient medically or biochemically (in the event of a distal cancer with copious vomiting). The fundamental aim of gastric cancer resection is for full excision of the primary lesion, the surrounding stomach and the relevant lymph nodes to an extent compatible with patient survival.

The location of the tumour in the stomach has a bearing on whether a total or partial gastrectomy is required, based on the need to achieve stomach clearance margins of 8–10 cm in the unstretched organ. These resection margins are required because tumour cells tend to spread in the submucosa of the stomach wall where they cannot be felt. Many surgeons advocate total gastrectomy for all gastric cancers whereas others favour a more limited approach for distal cancers because the healing and functional results may be better if a part of the upper stomach is retained.

Removal of the draining lymph nodes is essential in stomach cancer surgery because they are involved in this cancer in approximately 60% of Western patients and clearance of tumour cells in the lymph nodes improves the long-term outcome substantially. Lymph nodes around the stomach are divided into three sequential tiers: N1 nodes (around the stomach wall itself), N2 nodes (around the segmental arteries supplying the stomach and tumour) and N3 nodes (essentially deeper still). The location of these nodes is well documented and knowledge of them is essential to the surgeon, whose success depends on removing as many as possible.

Surgical resection of the stomach and the draining N1 nodes is called an R1 gastrectomy; if the N2 nodes are also removed en bloc with the specimen this becomes an R2 gastrectomy and usually involves removal of the peritoneum of the lesser sac, the greater and lesser omenta, and the pancreatic capsule, together with mobilization of the distal pancreas. An R3 resection goes further still, removing the spleen and distal pancreas, but this is associated with an increased morbidity that may not be outweighed by the ultimate benefit in most patients. The 'R' classification therefore refers to the extent of resection of the lymph node stations and is qualified descriptively by the extent of the stomach resection, e.g. R1 total gastrectomy, R2 subtotal gastrectomy, etc.

Once the stomach has been removed, reconstruction of the alimentary tract is achieved by mobilizing the small bowel, which is then free enough to join to the lower oesophagus or upper stomach (in the case of a distal gastrectomy). Failure of this anastomosis to heal is a notorious and major complication of this operation, with significant mortality.

Gastrectomy is a major operation with a very significant risk of complications. The overall mortality rate after it should be less than 5% but, in patients with advanced disease that cannot be removed by surgery, the mortality rate is very much higher at about 30%. Palliative gastrectomy is not therefore recommended.

As stomach cancer has a lethal tendency to spread directly across the peritoneal cavity (transcoelomic spread) in a manner often not detectable by CT or ultrasonography, many surgeons employ laparoscopy preoperatively to check against this possible spread and thus try to avoid an otherwise futile laparotomy for their patient.

Palliative surgery for gastric cancer is occasionally needed to relieve distressing symptoms of vomiting caused by obstruction or bleeding, but the less complex the level of surgery in these circumstances the better because the mortality is high.

For early gastric cancer a new treatment modality has recently been employed namely endoscopic submucosal resection (endoscopic SMR). In this the lesion is located endoscopically and a bleb of saline injected into the submucosa, causing the mucosa to rise into a polyp shape, which can then be ensnared and removed. This is applicable only to very early lesions and, if resection margins are involved histologically, formal surgical resection is required. It is rare in the UK to identify a patient who fulfils these criteria.

Postoperatively, patients who make a full recovery will need to have 3-monthly injections of vitamin B_{12} because the lack of a stomach prevents this vitamin from being absorbed enterally and anaemia would otherwise ensue. The patient will be able to eat small meals regularly and, with a good diet, will not suffer other nutritional disturbances. However, rarely will they become overweight.

If a splenectomy has been performed, patients will require immunization and may require long-term antibiotic prophylaxis against the risk of postsplenectomy sepsis, which is a serious but uncommon late complication of splenectomy. In addition, antithrombotic prophylaxis in the form of aspirin may be required for these patients.

Supplemental therapies

As with oesophageal cancer, knowledge of the TNM status of the tumour, based on all available evidence including histopathology, will allow staging of the tumour to be performed. As the stomach is such a large organ, assessment of nodal status is more complex because tumours at different sites drain into different N1 and N2 nodes, and staging is correspondingly a little more complex. However, established systems are in place and the staging of tumours may give a reasonable assessment of overall prognosis. It has been shown that, for tumours at high risk of relapse, survival benefit may be seen if adjuvant chemoradiotherapy is given after surgery and research is ongoing. Patients who have residual disease after surgery or those who develop recurrence may sometimes be offered chemotherapy but there is no evidence, as yet, that this affects life expectancy compared with no active treatment.

Prognosis

In the West, 90% of patients die within 5 years of diagnosis, whereas in the National Cancer Centre, Japan, 67% survive. The 5-year survival rate of patients undergoing surgery for early gastric cancer is greater than 90% but the results deteriorate with advancing stage of disease. If no lymph nodes are involved a 5-year survival rate of 60% might be expected, dropping to 25% if lymph nodes are involved.

Pancreatic cancer

In Britain and the USA, 100 patients with pancreatic cancer will present each year for each million of the population. The disease is rare below the age of 40 and 80% of cases occur in the 60- to 80-year age group. As with oesophageal and gastric cancer, men are more frequently affected.

Presentation

At least two-thirds of pancreatic cancers arise in the head of the pancreas and the most common presenting symptom is that of 'painless' obstructive jaundice. In this type of jaundice, which is caused by obstruction to the common bile duct, the jaundice is associated with darkened urine and a pale stool and is frequently accompanied by pruritus. There may be a palpable gallbladder on clinical examination (Courvoissier's sign). The term 'painless' refers to the lack of the colicky pain, which characterizes bile duct blockage caused by gallstones. However, a dull, vague, steady back pain is described by up to 70% of patients at the time of diagnosis, often radiating to or confined to the back; sometimes this is an ominous symptom signifying local invasion and irresectability. Anorexia, nausea and vomiting are often present and there is frequently a history of obvious weight loss. An episode of acute pancreatitis is sometimes the first presenting feature, and advanced cases may cause duodenal obstruction and persistent vomiting. Gastrointestinal bleeding is sometimes a late manifestation and is exacerbated in the presence of jaundice, as clotting abnormalities are common.

The remaining pancreatic tumours occur in the body and tail of the gland and these tumours tend to present late in their natural history, being mostly asymptomatic in the early stages, and recent-onset diabetes is present in 15% of cases. The presentation of these lesions tends to be as complications of secondary spread of disease or occasionally as a result of intestinal obstruction caused by direct invasion around the duodenum. Weight loss and paraneoplastic syndromes are common.

Investigations

The patient presenting with obstructive jaundice will undergo the following investigative pathway.

Blood tests

- Full blood count to assess for anaemia.
- Bioprofile to assess for signs of renal impairment (urea, creatinine and potassium) because jaundice itself may cause renal toxicity (the 'hepatorenal syndrome') and aggressive fluid management may be required to avert this problem.
- Liver function tests: in most patients the bilirubin will be raised as will alkaline phosphatase, but the level of transaminases will be relatively normal. The differential abnormalities of these measurements helps to confirm the nature of the jaundice.
- Clotting profile: the absorption of fat-soluble vitamins is impaired by the absence of bile in the intestine, caused by biliary obstruction. One of these is vitamin K, which has a short half-life and is essential for the clotting cascade. The prothrombin time (PTT) is therefore increased and such patients should be given parenteral vitamin K, especially as some form of invasive intervention will soon be needed.
- Tumour markers: the best marker for pancreatic cancer is serum Ca19-9, which has a sensitivity in diagnosing pancreatic cancer of 90%. However, values can be normal in the early stages of the disease and Ca19-9 is often raised simply by the presence of obstructive jaundice and may settle once the obstruction is relieved.

Radiology

Ultrasonography

This is the first-line investigation in the patient with obstructive jaundice because it confirms that the main bile duct and the intrahepatic ducts are dilated and therefore obstructed. It occasionally identifies the site and cause of the obstruction but, as the pancreatic head is not well seen on ultrasonography, this is not its primary purpose, and if the cause is not apparent then CT is indicated.

Computed tomography

It is essential that CT is performed before any intervention to the biliary tree because ERCP and percutaneous transhepatic cholangiography (PTC – see below) will obscure accurate interpretations of the scans. CT gives good views of the pancreatic head, allowing the diagnosis to be confirmed and, importantly, it will give invaluable information as to whether the tumour is operable. Occasionally no tumour is seen, but this is often the result of the tumour being very small and such patients may be those best suited to undergo surgery. The presence of liver metastases is usually best demonstrated by ultrasonography unless a dedicated liver CT scan is performed.

Endoscopic retrograde cholangiopancreatography

This procedure, usually performed under sedation, combines endoscopic and radiological techniques. Under sedation a side-viewing endoscope is introduced through the mouth into the duodenum, where the ampulla of Vater is identified, and a fine catheter is introduced through the endoscope into the bile duct. The site of obstruction may be seen by injecting contrast into the bile duct under radiological control and it is possible to introduce a plastic stent over the cannula and across the lesion, where it is left in place to allow the jaundice to drain. It is also possible to use metal stents as an alternative, but these cannot then be removed at a later date if surgery is contemplated. Sometimes, at ERCP it is seen that the obstruction is not the result of a cancer of the pancreatic head but rather of a cancer of the ampulla of Vater (ampullary carcinoma), for which the treatments are similar but for which the prognosis after treatment is better. Occasionally gallstones may be seen as the cause of the jaundice revising the diagnosis altogether and these can be removed immediately during ERCP.

Percutaneous transhepatic cholangiography

PTC is a technique whereby the liver is punctured via the skin on the abdomen using a fine needle, and then directed into one of the dilated bile ducts in the liver substance under radiological control. A catheter may then be passed along this into the major bile ducts and radiography will show the site and nature of the obstruction. Once performed, a stent may be deployed over this catheter and across the blockage. Alternatively, the catheter may be left in place to allow external biliary drainage as a temporizing manoeuvre.

Treatment options

Surgical excision offers the only chance of cure in pancreatic cancer. Unfortunately, only 10% of patients with cancer of the pancreatic head and less than 2% of those with carcinoma of the body and tail have lesions amenable to surgery at the time of presentation and some, otherwise eligible, patients will be medically unfit for such major surgery. For tumours to be considered resectable, there must be no evidence of spread beyond the pancreas or its immediate lymph nodes and there must be no involvement of the portal vein. Ideally the tumour should be less than 2 cm in diameter because larger tumours carry a worse prognosis. Some surgeons advocate a diagnostic laparoscopy to ensure that these criteria are fulfilled before proceeding to surgery.

Surgical procedures

Proximal pancreaticoduodenectomy (Whipple's operation)

This is the traditional and still the most favoured approach in which the distal stomach, the whole of the duodenum and the head of the pancreas are removed en bloc. This is a major undertaking and involvement of nearby vessels identified only at surgery may prevent completion of the operation. In addition, three major anastomoses are required (re-joining the stomach and the bile duct and the pancreatic duct to the small bowel separately). The latter two anastomoses have a reputation for being unreliable because they normally carry digestive secretions and failure to heal is a major complication. The operative mortality rate for this operation is in the order of 5–10%. An alternative version of this operation preserves the distal stomach and pylorus (the Longmire or pylorus-preserving proximal pancreaticoduodenectomy – PPPD). This procedure retains the entire stomach as a reservoir; as a result postgastrectomy complications are said to be lessened, but at a potential cost to the radicality of resection.

Distal pancreatectomy

This resection is indicated for lesions located in the body and tail of the gland and is almost always combined with splenectomy. It is usually performed for the rarer, slow-growing malignant tumours including cystadenocarcinoma and papillary–cystic neoplasm because the more common adenocarcinoma is rarely caught early enough for this to be an option.

Palliative treatment

Most patients are unsuitable for surgery and alternative strategies such as chemotherapy and radiotherapy are considered once the major symptoms of the disease are ameliorated.

Palliation is usually achieved by non-surgical methods and surgery is reserved for those in whom non-surgical palliation is not possible or in the circumstance where radical resectional surgery becomes impossible during the course of the operation.

The aims of palliation are to relieve jaundice, relieve or prevent duodenal obstruction, and ameliorate pain.

Jaundice is the major presenting symptom and in the inoperable patient may be treated by stenting either endoscopically or percutaneously. Plastic stents have a reputation for late blockage and usually only last 6 months before they need replacing. Metal stents, on the other hand, although more expensive are durable and do not need to be changed. Rarely, they may block as a result of tumour overgrowth in which case a second stent is occasionally necessary.

Duodenal obstruction occurs in only 10% of patients with inoperable pancreatic head cancer and usually requires surgical bypass because stents for the duodenum are still experimental. When treated in isolation, duodenal obstruction may often be bypassed using laparoscopic surgery, but, if this is a presenting complaint with jaundice, laparotomy and 'triple' bypass are sometimes preferred, in which the small bowel is anastomosed to the stomach, the bile duct and to itself to relieve duodenal and biliary obstruction simultaneously.

Additional treatments

The value of adjuvant and neoadjuvant therapy in the treatment of pancreatic cancer is much less well defined than for stomach and oesophageal cancer, with current results suggesting marginal benefit. However, various combinations are currently under evaluation and most patients with locally advanced lesions will be eligible for entry into postoperative clinical trials to try to improve this situation. There is a vogue for additional radiotherapy in the USA, which is not generally shared in the UK, and further results are anticipated as to the best approach. Palliative chemotherapy may be considered in patients with advanced, non-resectable or recurrent disease based on the patient's general well-being.

Duodenal cancers

Adenocarcinoma of the duodenum is a rare malignancy accounting for 5% of periampullary tumours. Many of these tumours arise in pre-existing villous adenomas, especially in patients with familial polyposis coli, in whom primary duodenal carcinoma is the second most common malignancy. These cancers are rare and resection is along similar lines and with similar results as for pancreatic cancer.

Gallbladder cancer

Gallbladder cancer is a rare gastrointestinal malignancy with approximately 6600 new cases diagnosed each year in the USA. The peak incidence is in the seventh decade, with women affected three to four times more commonly than men and the cancer is almost invariably associated with the presence of gall-stones. As some patients with gallbladder cancer present with the clinical picture of acute cholecystitis, or empyema of the gallbladder, it is often recognized during investigation or treatment for gallstone-type symptoms. In many, it is detected incidentally during elective gallbladder surgery for stones.

In patients presenting with acute cholecystitis, the disease is usually incurable at the time of presentation and palliative chemotherapy or localized radiotherapy is usually advised. The incidental finding of gallbladder cancer on histology after routine elective surgery presents a difficult decision. Some have advocated an aggressive approach mandating a full laparotomy, removal of all surrounding tissue (usually involving a partial hepatectomy) and excision of the port sites if the original cholecystectomy was performed laparoscopically. If the patient is not fit enough for this or if histology is otherwise favourable, an observant policy will be preferred. It is not uncommon for such patients to re-present with a second primary bile duct cancer (cholangiocarcinoma) and it is felt that there may be a field change in the bile duct mucosa, with these types of tumour predisposing to multiple sites of unstable cells.

Prognosis

Except for early, incidentally detected, gallbladder cancer most centres report consistently unsatisfactory results even with radical surgery performed. The overall 5-year survival rate is less than 5% and few patients survive more than 1 year when they present with advanced disease.

Bile duct tumours (cholangiocarcinomas)

Bile duct adenocarcinomas are uncommon tumours, which usually present with obstructive jaundice in much the same way as pancreatic tumours. Approximately half arise in the distal common bile duct and, if they arise in the terminal 1 cm, are referred to as periampullary tumours along with ampullary cancers of Vater. The remaining bile duct cancers arise in the upper biliary tree and, if they involve the confluence of left and right hepatic ducts, are known as 'Klatskin' tumours. Bile duct cancer is most common in the seventh decade but about 20% occur in patients aged under 45 years. These tumours tend to spread locally into the surrounding tissues and most become inoperable because of this. Some are also found to be multifocal within the biliary tree.

Treatment is ideally by surgical resection; however, only 15–20% of lesions are amenable to surgery and lower tumours are more likely to be resectable than upper tumours. Lower bile duct cancers are treated by radical surgical resection, using the Whipple operation. A 30% 5-year survival rate is possible after such surgery and this compares favourably with the results obtained by the Whipple operation for pancreatic cancer. Upper bile duct tumours are rarely resectable, but those arising within the liver itself may occasionally be removed with a partial hepatectomy. Experience with radical resection of the upper bile ducts, total hepatectomy and liver transplantation has not proved encouraging and is not currently advocated. For non-resectable tumours, palliation with a combination of stents, chemotherapy and radiotherapy is usually appropriate and some patients survive for long periods after this. Metal stents are generally preferred because bile duct cancers tend to be slower growing than pancreatic cancers and the metal stents are more durable. Recent interest has focused on the use of endoluminal brachytherapy with the insertion of a radioactive source into the bile duct itself. This treatment appears to give reasonably good local control and experience with some of the more modern chemotherapeutic agents is also proving encouraging in the treatment of these difficult tumours.

Chemoradiotherapy

Patients with bile duct and gallbladder cancers are rarely suitable to be considered for surgery. Chemotherapy (gemcitabine and cisplatin) is often offered, occasionally with remarkable success. Some patients may survive for considerable periods of time with biliary carcinoma with or without chemotherapy.

Primary liver cancer

The majority of liver cancer in the UK is secondary disease, most frequently from a primary colorectal cancer. However, primary cancers of the liver do occur and are hepatocellular carcinomas (HCCs). In the UK this is a rare disease but in other parts of the world it is not and primary HCC is possibly the most common intra-abdominal cancer worldwide. This is because of a very high incidence in the Far East, China and Africa. The explanation lies in the aetiology and the major cause of HCC is thought to be cirrhosis from chronic active hepatitis resulting from viral diseases such as hepatitis B and C, which are highly prevalent in those societies but less so in ours.

The diagnosis is made on radiological appearances (in the West) and by the finding of a raised α-fetoprotein tumour marker in the serum. Biopsy is reserved for patients whose disease is unresectable because the act of biopsy technically renders the tumour inoperable by virtue of seeding tumour cells along the biopsy track. About 10% of primary liver tumours are resectable and one subtype – the fibrolamellar type, often seen in younger women – responds very well to surgical therapy. Irresectability is not always the result of very advanced tumour or multifocality, but most often is precluded by the diseased state of the surrounding cirrhotic liver which, when left, would provide insufficient liver reserve to permit survival after resection of the primary lesion.

Chemoradiotherapy has no current role to play in the treatment of HCC and indeed most conventional chemotherapeutic agents are metabolized by the liver and cannot be given where there is limited liver reserve.

Local control of a primary hepatic tumour may sometimes be achieved by the insertion of a probe into the centre of the tumour and delivering local tissue damage. Such damage may be achieved using cryotherapy (local tissue freezing probe) or by microwave or radiofrequency ablation delivered percutaneously under radiological or ultrasound guidance or on occasion via a laparoscope (key hole surgery). A more novel method is to starve the tumour of blood using selective arterial embolisation, but all these treatments are currently considered inferior to surgical resection where possible.

The role of the nurse practitioner

Cancers of the upper GI tract form an aggressive group of tumours, which tend to present late in their natural history and for which major surgical procedures are needed, often with poor outcomes. Not all patients will recover fully from illness and many must learn to cope with permanent health changes, which may well include changes within the family role. In many instances the family is a vital part of the support mechanism in the patient's recovery and may need support themselves in later stages of the disease process.

Depression may bring about additional symptoms of anorexia and insomnia, or behavioural effects such as social withdrawal. Pain from progressive cancer is usually constant and debilitating, but may be relieved by increased and vigilant pain management or the application of special techniques such as pressure vibration and/or massage. Discomfort may be caused by physical irritation resulting from dry skin or jaundice, and once again pain management and appropriate medication should ease these symptoms. Many other symptoms may lead to discomfort and incapacity such as fatigue, constipation, malnutrition and dehydration; however, they are not discussed in this chapter because they have been extensively considered elsewhere in this book.

The NP must maintain an overview of the patient's progress and act as a resource for information. Patients for whom palliative care is the option may require relief of symptoms, which in the case of dysphagia or biliary obstruction may involve stent insertion.

Percutaneous endoscopic gastrostomy

It is important to identify patients who need feeding tubes before they become nutritionally depleted. Patients with upper GI disease may require a feeding tube because of impaired swallowing or immediately after surgery of the upper GI tract.

When the patient cannot ingest, chew or swallow food, but is able to digest and absorb nutrients, a feeding tube is placed into the stomach (gastrostomy). This is a long, hollow, flexible catheter inserted into the stomach through the skin in the upper left quadrant of the abdomen. This may be inserted directly through a surgical incision but, if endoscopic access into the stomach is possible, percutaneous endoscopic gastrostomy (PEG) is the preferred option because it may be inserted with minimally invasive techniques and under simple sedation, thus reducing the need for general anaesthetic and surgical wound.

For long-term feeding, a gastrostomy tube may be replaced with a skin level device, commonly referred to as a button. The entry site is flush with the skin, making it neat and less conspicuous than a gastrostomy tube.

Coordinating care

It is important that the nurse practitioner acts as a coordinator in the care of patients with upper GI cancers as their needs are multiple and quite often the prognosis poor. Appendix II identifies some areas of care in which the nurse practitioner should be involved. Ultimately, the aim is for a seamless service, and the exchange of relevant, accurate information between primary and secondary care services will facilitate this requirement.

Conclusions

This chapter has aimed to identify some of the complexities involved in the care of patients with upper GI cancer. As has been illustrated, decisions around appropriate diagnosis and treatment techniques are not simple or at times clearly defined. The patient should be supported through investigative processes, which may be complex. Many of the treatments offered in upper GI cancer disease are harsh and debilitating, with an unknown prognosis, so social, psychological and symptom support will be extensively required to this group of patients.

References

Barrett NR (1950) Chronic peptic ulcer of the oesophagus and 'oesophagitis'. British Journal of Surgery 38: 175-182.

Gordon M (1987) Nursing Diagnosis: Process and application. New York : McGraw-Hill.

Lewis I (1947) Surgical treatment of carcinoma of the oesophagus with special reference to a new operation for growths of the middle third. British Journal of Surgery 34: 18-31.

McKeown KC (1981) Resection of mid-oesophageal carcinoma with oesophagogastric anastomosis. World Journal of Surgery 5: 517-525.

Muir C, Waterhouse J, Mack T, Powell J, Whelan S (1987) Cancer Incidence in Five Continents, vol 6. IARC Scientific Publication no. 88. Lyon: IARC.

Parkin DM, Pisani P, Ferlay J (1993) Estimates of the worldwide incidence of eigh-
    teen major cancers in 1985. International Journal of Cancer.
Wilson-Barnett J, Carrigy A (1978) Factors influencing patients' emotional reac-
    tions to hospitalization. Journal of Advanced Nursing. 3: 221–229.

Appendix I

Staging systems

Oesophageal tumours

T category

T1	– tumour localized to the mucosa or submucosa
T2	– tumour invading the muscularis propria
T3	– tumour invading the adventitia
T4	– tumour invading other structures

N category

N0	– no regional metastases
N1	– regional lymph node metastases

M category

M0	– no distant metastases
M1	– distant metastases

Staging system – oesophagus

Stage 0	Tis, N0, M0
Stage I	T1, N0, M0
Stage IIa	T2, N0, M0; T3, N0, M0
Stage IIb	T1, N1, M0; T2, N1, M0
Stage III	T3,4, N1, M0; T4, N0, M0
Stage IV	M1

Gastric tumours

T category

T0	– no evidence of primary tumour
Tis	– carcinoma *in situ*; intraepithelial tumour only
T1	– tumour invades lamina propria or submucosa
T2	– tumour invades muscularis propria (T2a) or subserosa (T2b)

| T3 | – tumour penetrates the serosa without invasion of surrounding structures |
| T4 | – tumour invades adjacent structures |

N category

N0	– no regional metastases
N1	– metastases in perigastric lymph nodes within 3 cm of the tumour
N2	– metastases in perigastric lymph nodes > 3 cm from the tumour or in any level 2 lymph nodes

M category

| M0 | No distant metastases |
| M1 | Distant metastases |

Staging system – stomach

Stage I	T1, N0, M0 (Ia); T1, N1, M0 (Ia); T2, N0, M0; (Ib)
Stage II	T1, N2, M0; T2, N1,M0; T3, N0, M0
Stage III	T2, N2, M0; T4, N0, M0; T3, N1, M0 T3, N2, M0, T4, N1, M0
Stage IV	T4, N2, M0; any T, any N, M1

Pancreatic tumours

T category

T1	Limited to the pancreas. (T1a < 2cm, T1b > 2cm)
T2	Extends directly into duodenum, bile duct, peripancreatic tissues
T3	Extends directly to stomach, spleen, colon, adjacent large vessels

N category

| N0 | No regional metastases |
| N1 | Regional metastases |

M category

| M0 | No distant metastases |
| M1 | Distant metastases |

Pancreatic tumour staging

Stage 1	T1-2, N0, M0
Stage 2	T3, N0, M0
Stage 3	T1-3, N1, M0
Stage 4	T1-3, N0-1, M1

Appendix II

Promoting research and using best practice in upper GI care

The nurse practitioner will:

- Provide clinical leadership to other nursing staff, acting as a resource for education and clinical expertise
- Be familiar with current clinical research protocols, relevant investigations and procedures involved in the diagnosis and management of gastrointestinal disease
- Be competent in discussing options and surgical procedures, in addition to chemotherapy and radiotherapy treatments
- Identify skills and practices that can be applied to shape local and national policy to promote better care overall
- Participate in clinical case conferences
- Review and develop patient information systems
- Acknowledge recommendations from national bodies
- Participate in research projects
- Write and monitor standards of care
- Participate in service reviews
- Lead on the development, implementation and evaluation of integrated care pathways for patients with upper gastrointestinal disease
- Provide education and counselling
- Provide an educational resource to other health professionals
- Develop educational packages and coordinate educational programmes
- Assist in the development of information services for upper gastrointestinal disease
- Collaborate with higher education and post-registration programmes
- Act as a resource for local support groups.

Chapter 6
Cancer of the lower gastrointestinal tract: colon and rectal cancer

MANDIE BULMER AND GRAEME DUTHIE

Colon and rectal cancers are currently among the most common cancers in the Western World. Coming second only to lung cancer in the whole population, and to breast cancer in women, as a cause of cancer-associated mortality, although lung cancer in women is rising. There will be some 32 000 new diagnoses of colorectal cancer made this year and subsequently 50% of these patients will succumb to their disease. As survival is stage specific, in theory early recognition of the signs and symptoms leading to the appropriate diagnosis should incur some survival advantage. The problem is that many of the symptoms and signs of colon and rectal cancer are very non-specific and the natural history of the disease suggests that the development of a cancer through the normal sequence of mucosa to polyp to cancer may take in excess of 10 years. We can, however, split the instances of colon and rectal cancer into two groups – genetic and sporadic – the split being roughly 15% and 85%, respectively.

Cancers with a genetic basis, the so-called familial cancers, and perhaps those that occur in patients with ulcerative colitis and Crohn's disease, can be predicted and identified reasonably reliably with the appropriate family or disease history. There is the potential that this high-risk group could be screened to good effect. It is only by giving support and information that effective communication between families can be maintained. Care should be taken when screening this group of patients to ensure that their journey through endoscopy is friendly and open. The patients who fall within this group will require extra support and understanding. The treatment they receive will be reported to other family members and may dictate whether or not other family members attend for screening. In addition, these patients become well known to the team and sometimes provide an education resource for those newly diagnosed with familial disorders. It is essential that patients are aware of the risk without being overwhelmed by fear of the disease. A good screening programme is effective only if used by the patients deemed to be at risk.

Sporadic cancers arise in a population that has no known family history of colon and/or rectal cancer. This is a large group, where there has to be a reliance on patient symptomatology for diagnosis because the signs and symptoms of bowel cancer are relatively vague. It is quite common for presentation to be very late and, as prognosis is stage related, it follows that there is a relatively high mortality from this disease. Detection relies not only on patients recognizing the symptoms and visiting their general practitioner, but also on the GP making an early referral to a colorectal consultant. The best chance of reducing the incidence of colon and rectal cancer is to introduce generalized population screening programmes. Such screening would be required either to detect sporadic or genetic cancers that have a better long-term prognosis at an earlier stage, or to detect adenomatous polyps that are known to be a major risk factor in carcinogenesis.

There is, however, a third group of patients that should be considered when looking at the incidence of colon and rectal cancers; this is the group of patients who develop cancer of the anus. This group accounts for a smaller percentage of the patients that we treat – around 1–5%. Anal cancer is a known complication in patients who are diagnosed as having human papilloma virus (HPV), especially types 16 and 18, and these patients may also have had cancers of the cervix, vagina and vulval area. These patients are at high risk of developing an anal cancer and this area should be screened at regular intervals, using a colposcope.

The development of colon and rectal cancer from normal bowel through adenomatous polyp to a cancer is now relatively well documented and this process is known to take anything from 10 to 15 years. The underlying chromosomal changes that are associated with carcinogenesis are relatively well known in this process. It seems likely that it is an interaction between the patient genotype and the environmentally affected phenotype that is crucial in the development of sporadic colorectal cancer.

There have been many theories about the effect of fibre, fats and other dietary components, including red meat, etc., as well as suggestions related to known hazards such as smoking. It is likely that, as our knowledge of the human genetic code improves, a higher proportion of cancers will be ascribed to an underlying genetic or chromosomal cause that may be identifiable in the laboratory. This is, however, many years off and so detection of these cases will rely on case presentation.

We know that the cardinal sign – 'a change in bowel habit', in either direction from normal towards either diarrhoea or constipation – can herald a sinister diagnosis, as can rectal bleeding. The instance of these symptoms within the normal population is, however, very high and if we were to investigate fully all patients with these symptoms, the resource implications would probably be insurmountable. There is no doubt that these symptoms, coupled with signs of systemic illness such as anaemia, weight loss, tiredness and/or lethargy, should raise a high index of suspicion, and patients presenting in this manner should be rapidly investigated to exclude large bowel cancers. Similarly, those patients with persistent, rather than transitory, symptoms are also more likely to have some significant pathology, so continuous bleeding for more than 6 weeks, or a continuous change in bowel habit over the same period, should also lead to urgent investigation. The incidence of malignancy in these patients is much higher. Many will be aware of the guidelines that have been announced in the UK to help primary and secondary care physicians identify patients at high risk and speed them though the system. These guidelines are listed in Table 6.1. This is not exclusive and other presentations may also warrant urgent investigation.

It is worth noting that there is a tendency for right- and left-sided cancers to differ in their presentation. The bowel contents that exit the terminal ileum into the right side of the large bowel are much more fluid than on the left side of the colon and rectum; here it is much more solid as a result of water extraction from the stool content. Simple physics dictates that, for a lesion to obstruct in the right side of the colon, it must almost totally obstruct the large bowel lumen to stop fluid flow. An obstruction in the left side of the colon is likely to happen with much less luminal obstruction because of the solid nature of faecal material. This is partly why cancers in the right side of the colon

Table 6.1 Urgent patient guidelines (2-week wait)

Patients being referred must fulfil one or more of the following five criteria (criteria 1 and 2 relate to patients > 60 years of age; criteria 3, 4 and 5 relate to patients of any age)

1. Persistent rectal bleeding without anal symptoms (soreness, discomfort, itching, lumps, prolapses, pain, etc.)
2. Change of bowel habit to looser stools and/or increased urgency of defecation persistent for 6 weeks
3. Rectal bleeding AND a change of bowel habit to looser stools and/or increased frequency of defecation persistent for 6 weeks
4. A palpable rectal or right-sided abdominal mass
5. Iron deficiency anaemia WITHOUT an obvious cause: men Hb < 11 g/dl; women Hb < 10 g/dl

Department of Health website (www.doh.gov.uk/pub/docs/doh/guidelines.pdf).

notoriously present late. It should be remembered that patients who present with small bowel symptoms may have caecal or ascending colon obstruction lesions, which cause small, rather than large, bowel symptoms.

Rectal bleeding is a relatively vague sign. Many people at some point in their life have a show of blood from acute fissures or minor piles, which is clearly self-limiting; without any other symptoms that suggest colonic disease, this needs little further investigation. There is evidence that rectal bleeding presenting with anal symptoms is a very poor indicator of major colonic pathology. Patients presenting with dark as opposed to bright red rectal bleeding have a much higher incidence of significant colonic pathology, and these patients probably warrant urgent investigation. As noted previously, patients who present with large bowel symptoms in conjunction with systemic signs of disease are likely to be at a later stage of diagnosis, as are those with a palpable mass in the abdomen.

There is a general lack of awareness of colon and rectal symptoms in the UK and Europe. As with breast cancer, considerable improvements may be made in stage of presentation and therefore prognosis by a concerted educational effort for the population. It seems likely that there would be considerable scope for a practitioner to operate under such circumstances, promoting colorectal awareness within an area either through local media presentations or presentation via primary care services.

Screening

Effective screening of the patients that fall within these groups is essential if we are to diagnose colon and rectal cancer in its early stages. The World Health Organization (WHO) has identified the principles of a good screening programme.

The disease being screened for:

- must have a significant morbidity or mortality
- must be sufficiently common to make screening worthwhile
- should have a premalignant phase (this is accepted as the adenomatous polyp).

The tests used to screen for the disease should:

- be sufficiently acceptable for large numbers of the population to cooperate with, and therefore use, a screening programme
- have a very low risk of any morbidity and mortality.

Of course, any screening programme has to be financially viable and there is good evidence that there would be appropriate financial advantages to screening for colon and rectal cancer, but this depends on certain assumptions. The 'gold standard' for large bowel investigation is colonoscopy; however, this would prove far too expensive as a screening test used in the general population. Faecal occult blood (FOB) testing has been shown to improve morbidity and mortality in relation to colon and rectal cancer outcome and to downstage cancers at the point of presentation and discovery with a resultant improvement in the prognosis. The problem is that the test is so sensitive that it potentially results in a large number of false positives, with a subsequent large number of colonoscopies giving relatively low yields. In addition, there is the question of patient compliance with the drug and dietary restrictions associated with FOB testing and the necessity for returning faecal samples on test strips to the laboratory over many years. The increased anxiety among the population as a result of the false positives also needs to be considered.

We know that 70% of colon and rectal cancers are distal to the splenic flexure and therefore it seems logical that a significant amount of cancer is within the range of the flexible sigmoidoscope from a detection point of view. There are currently large trials going on in the UK into flexible sigmoidoscopic screening, and the outcome is eagerly awaited. One problem, if this is developed further, is the resource of highly trained personnel undertaking large numbers of flexible sigmoido-scopies. With the pressure on endoscopic services already very high, to take on this flexible sigmoidoscopic screening would require extra personnel resources. The only realistic place from which this could come in the long term is endoscopically trained nurse practitioners; in fact there might be significant patient benefits from this. Such nurse practitioners would have more time and possibly we could admit that they would take a much more holistic approach to the patient. The colorectal cancer screening could also produce the opportunity for other health benefits provided by these practitioners.

Of the 30% of remaining cancers, which occur proximal to the splenic flexure, many have some incidental lesion in the colon distal to the splenic flexure; this implies that colono-scopic evaluation should be undertaken, e.g. small adenomatous polyps and some of these right-sided lesions are detected by default at subsequent evaluation. It should also be noted that those with hereditary non-polyposis-type cancers and other autonomic dominant cancers have a preponderance to a right-sided lesion; these would therefore make up a number of the right-sided cases that have the potential to be missed with flexi-ble sigmoidoscopic screening. It is hoped, however, that these would be caught on an appropriate high-risk screening programme. There is some evidence to suggest that compliance may be a problem in colon and rectal cancer screening and nurse practitioners may also have a useful role in this aspect of screening promotion.

High-risk screening

There is, without doubt, evidence that screening should be undertaken in patients who can be identified as having a high risk of developing colon and rectal cancers, e.g. those with a family history of familial adenomatous polyposis (FAP), heredi-tary non-polyposis colorectal cancer (HNPCC), other dominant cancer syndromes, long-term ulcerative colitis and Crohn's disease. These patients probably form between 10% and 20% of all cancer presentations, and in many cases potential patients and their families are easily identified with a simple family history. It therefore seems logical that these patients should be offered appropriate and regular colonic screening and a genetic assessment, with a view to screening other areas where cancers affect patients with these syndromes. The resource for screening these patients would be of higher priority than screening for sporadic cancer, in that they would all require full colonic screening on a very regular basis. However, it would seem that the yield in financial terms of lives saved would far exceed the costs. Perhaps, in the future, there may be a role for nurse practitioners interested in family cancer syndromes and those interested in endoscopy to take on the screening of these high-risk individuals, although clearly there would have to be an adequate move towards training them in colonoscopic surveillance.

The easiest of all the genetic high-risk groups to identify are those with FAP. It seems likely, in the very near future, that appropriate genetic testing will be generally available for this and therefore the role of accurate colonoscopic surveillance and prophylactic surgery may become much more targeted. The other high-risk group that is readily identifiable is the group known as HNPCC. This is a slight misnomer because these patients do go through a polyp-to-cancer sequence, albeit accelerated compared with the normal sporadic sequence. It was named 'hereditary non-polyposis' to distinguish it from familial adenomatous polyposis. This group of patients used to be identified as having Lynch syndrome; they can be divided into two groups based on the other cancers associated with the bowel cancers within the family. In essence, however, although bowel cancer predominates in both these groups, families also present with ovarian or uterine cancers, urinary tract cancers, other gastrointestinal tract cancers or pancreatic cancers. Although the incidence of these cancers is much lower than colon and rectal cancer in this group, patients who are identified as having HNPCC will require screening for all these cancers as part of a high-risk screening programme. The definition of HNPCC is known as the 'Amsterdam criteria', which are recorded in Table 6.2. There is currently some discussion in the literature that these criteria are perhaps too strict and some of the other families exhibiting dominant patterns of cancer heredity should also be included. This is an area that is certainly worthy of further reading, but there is no space available in this text to explore it in greater detail. Other identifiable syndromes include Gardner's syndrome and the Peutz–Jeghers syndrome. There is also recognition of an association with hereditary breast cancer

Table 6.2 Amsterdam criteria (Burke et al., 1997)

Three relatives affected with colorectal cancer

One has to be a first-degree relative

One has to be under the age of 50 years

Disease has to occur over two generations

Familial adenomatous polyposis has to be excluded

Modifications to the criteria

Colorectal cancer diagnosed before the age of 40 years

Other cancers may replace colorectal cancer such as endometrial, stomach, urinary tract, ovarian or biliary tract (at least one must be colorectal cancer)

through the *BRCA* genes; there is therefore some logic in maintaining the history records of both colorectal and breast cancer patients together so that these connections become obvious.

Although there are these genetically identifiable syndromes, there are also clearly a number of patients in whom cancers seem to run in the family, although they do not conform to these noted patterns. Identification of family patterns that represent autosomal dominant inheritance remains important. Perhaps one of the major roles for nurse practitioners involved with the colorectal cancer service can be family history identification using each new patient that presents with cancer as a proband for the records. The risks within the families relate to the number, age and degree of relatives involved and these can be represented with the risks declared in Table 6.3.

Table 6.3 Lifetime risks of colorectal cancer in relative of affected patients (the Lovett table)

Risk definition	Risk estimate
Population risk	1 in 50
One first-degree relative affected, diagnosed >45 years old	1 in 17
One first- and one second-degree relative affected, diagnosed >45 years old	1 in 12
One first-degree relative diagnosed <45 years old	1 in 10
Two first-degree relatives affected	1 in 6
Three first-degree relatives affected (dominant pedigree)	1 in 2

From Houston et al. (1990).

For many years there has been a known association of colon and rectal cancer with long-standing ulcerative colitis and Crohn's disease. Although recently the risks associated with the development of cancer in long-term sufferers have been reduced somewhat, these risks are still real and certainly warrant inclusion of these patients in a high-risk group. The evidence pointing to high risks is mainly in those patients with a history of panproctocolitis rather than local distal colitis, and in those who have had this for a period in excess of 10 years. It seems reasonable that patients who fit these criteria are screened colonoscopically on a yearly basis, because cancers in this group of patients tend to develop rapidly and also tend to have a preponderance to the right side of the colon.

Adenomatous polyps

Many patients are referred for investigation and a proportion of these will have polyps either removed with snares or destroyed using diathermy. As a result of the known adenoma-to-carcinoma sequence, these patients must therefore be considered as having been at risk of developing colon or rectal cancer, although the incidence of polyps is higher than the incidence of cancer and therefore not every patient may have gone on to develop neoplastic disease. This has implications for the continued follow-up of these patients because of the risk. There is no doubt that the follow-up should be colonoscopical if at all possible, because a number of these patients will require further polyp intervention and regular barium assessment will lead to excessive doses of irradiation. A small number of these patients will fall into some of the higher-risk groups already discussed. However, the vast majority are represented within a sporadic group, and these patients, having had a polyp removed at diagnosis, may or may not develop further polyps. It therefore seems rational that these patients should have some sort of sensible follow-up policy to detect and eliminate adenomatous polyps and reduce the long-term risks of cancer.

Standard practice currently dictates that patients who have a diagnosis of an adenomatous polyp undergo colonoscopy yearly, with all polyps being removed until the colon is clear at the subsequent year's follow-up. As a result of the known prolonged adenoma–carcinoma sequence in sporadic cancer, it is then reasonable that the polyp screening interval may be expanded as standard practice. At the moment it expands to an initial 3-year assessment after a clear colon and, provided that assessment is clear, further assessment can continue at 5-yearly intervals. A ceiling is usually put at age 75 or 80 years for routine follow-up; thereafter follow-up is determined by symptomatic presentation.

Investigations

Many patients who present to the colorectal outpatients do so with a fear that they have bowel cancer. The role of the assessor in the outpatients' clinic is a vital one. A detailed history should be taken from the patient, including a family history. Abdominal examination should be undertaken and the rectum and anus evaluated digitally and using rigid sigmoidoscopy. The investigation of symptomatic patients can be divided into those with symptoms but without a confirmed diagnosis, and those with a confirmed diagnosis of colon or rectal cancer. These are dealt with separately below. In patients with signs and symptoms suggestive of colon and rectal cancer, the question arises as to the rationale for the investigation of the large bowel. There is no doubt that the gold standard assessment is colonoscopy because this allows not only visualization of the whole of the large bowel but also biopsy or polypectomies as appropriate. Colonoscopy does, however, have a number of associated risks, including bowel perforation and haemorrhage, and patients must be warned that surgical intervention may be necessary in these cases. The incidence of perforation and bleeding probably runs at about 1:1000 but, as these complications are potentially life threatening, even this level of risk should be discussed with the patient.

Colonoscopy is an investigation that is successful in varying percentages of patients. Many literature reports give the success rate of complete colonoscopy at between 90% and 98%, but there is a general feeling from the gastroenterological community that real rates are probably lower than this – somewhere between 75% and 90%. We therefore have to be able to audit the quality of colonoscopy. The gold standard for this is terminal ileal intubation and biopsy that leaves no doubt of complete colonoscopy. However, the cost and time of intubating the terminal ileum may reduce throughput on endoscopic lists, such that it becomes non-viable as a routine auditing tool. Others have used vision of appendiceal orifices, ileocaecal valve and right iliac fossa indentation but these are all less reliable than terminal ileal biopsy. More recently, clips have been applied to the caecal pole and patients have had a radiograph within 30 minutes of colonoscopy, when the colon is still full of air and the position of the clip can be readily identified. Clearly, any or all of these audit tools can be used but it is essential, in a dedicated colonoscopy unit, that some degree of audit is undertaken on a regular basis to ensure the continuing high quality of investigation.

It is also now essential with the Joint Advisory Group on Gastrointestinal Endoscopy (JAG) regulations that only suitably qualified personnel are allowed to perform colonoscopy without supervision (JAG, 1999). Failure to complete diagnostic colonoscopy should result in a further attempt, if failure was the result of poor bowel preparation or some other technical reason that would suggest a future successful colonoscopy; otherwise completion of the investigation should be with a barium enema. This should be considered first if there have been difficulties as a result of persistent looping of the scope or because of a very long colon.

Without colonoscopy facilities, double-contrast barium enema studies are clearly the next best choice for investigation of the large bowel. There are, however, limitations with this examination, which occur especially in the rectum where the ampulla is filled with the retaining balloon and rectal lesions can be missed. There is also difficulty in interpreting the sigmoid colon or the transverse loop because of overlying barium-filled loops obscuring the detail. It is now accepted that a barium enema alone, or combination with a rigid sigmoidoscopy, is an inadequate investigation of the large bowel. A barium enema must be combined with flexible sigmoidoscopy, which must achieve the splenic flexure and be of diagnostic value. Research has shown that a barium enema and flexible sigmoidoscopy performed in tandem are just as effective as screening the colon. Flexible sigmoidoscopy can be equally well performed by a nurse endoscopist or a doctor (Hughes et al., 1999).

There is, however, still a role for the flexible sigmoidoscope alone as a diagnostic tool. There are many patients who, on referral, can be identified as having a low risk of significant pathology, e.g. anyone under 45 with a single episode of bright-red bleeding, with no systemic signs or illness and no personal or family history of polyps or cancer. This group may well warrant flexible sigmoidoscopy complete to the splenic flexure as a simple investigation, to obviate the need for full assessment of the large bowel if they are otherwise asymptomatic. Clearly these patients and their primary care physicians do need to be warned that the large bowel investigations are incomplete and that, if symptoms return or become persistent, they should return promptly for full bowel investigation.

Despite radiological or endoscopic advancement, there are some patients in whom both will fail. Computed tomography (CT) is the investigation of choice to exclude large bowel lesions under these circumstances. The increasing use of virtual colonoscopy with spiral CT may in due course alter our investigative plans; however, there are still problems with both the resolution of CT colonoscopy and resources in relation to interpretation of the scans. In addition, patients showing up positive on CT will need colonoscopic assessment which will probably mean very little difference to the colonoscopy services in the long run.

It is also appropriate to undertake more general investigations of patients presenting with colorectal signs and symptoms. These vary from simply weighing patients for comparison with previously known weights to ascertain weight loss, through routine urine analysis, full blood counts to determine any degree of anaemia and biochemical profiles assessing liver function, to more specific tests associated with gastrointestinal disease. Inflammatory bowel disease uses C-reactive protein (CRP) as a marker and, along with this, the tumour markers carcinoembryonic antigen (CEA), Ca19.9 and Ca125 should also be routinely tested in patients with large bowel symptoms.

Diagnosis and support

The main aim of intensive screening is to arrive at a conclusive diagnosis. It is at the start of screening that extra information is important to the patient. Time taken in the outpatients department for an explanation of the need for further investigations and the importance of effective bowel preparation will ensure that the patient is correctly prepared when attending for screening. The roles of the nurse practitioner and radiology and endoscopy nursing staff are vital in the dissemination of this information, which increases the compliance and attendance at endoscopy and radiology by well-prepared patients and reduces the waste of resources from missed appointments, and failed investigations resulting from poor bowel preparation.

Once diagnosed, colon and rectal cancer falls into four main areas for treatment: the right hemicolon, left hemicolon, rectum and anal canal. It should be noted that the period of investigation is an anxious time for the patient and they will require support and information during this period. The role of the nurse practitioner is effective in providing a point of contact for support and information; a rapport can be established that will last throughout the patient treatment episode. This episode could be short, if the colon is clear, or more lengthy and last throughout colorectal cancer diagnosis, treatment and follow-up.

There is always considerable pressure from patients to get on and resect the cancer as soon as possible. Although this is completely understandable, it is important that time is taken to consider the surgery and accurately stage the disease so that the best and most appropriate operation can be undertaken in an attempt for cure. Most patients and their relatives attending the outpatients remember very little of the consultation after a diagnosis of cancer is given. Although it is important that the need for surgery, with its morbidity and mortality, is discussed with the patient at this point, and also the possible need for a temporary or permanent stoma, it is extremely useful to be able to counsel the patient further. The nurse practitioner is able to ensure that the patients are fully informed because their information requirements develop over the ensuing days and weeks. In the majority of cases, between 2 and 6 weeks will pass between giving the diagnosis and the actual surgery. During this time, staging procedures such as CT or magnetic resonance imaging (MRI) will be performed to evaluate the pelvis and liver, and further diagnostic procedures such as completion barium enemas or colonoscopies are performed.

The nursing involvement with the patient begins well before admission to hospital. Care of the patient is the responsibility of the multidisciplinary team, with each team member having a defined role. Information is essential to help the patient cope with the examinations and investigations that will be undertaken. This information needs to be delivered to the patient in a manner that he or she can comprehend. Honesty is important if the patient is to trust the team members. It is our policy to inform the patient of all the results as they become available. In this preoperative period, time is spent with the consultant and the nurse practitioner to discuss the findings of the investigations and the impact that these findings will have on the future treatment plan. There is no doubt that there is a significant role to play, during this intervening time, by the nurse practitioner acting as a counsellor, information resource and perhaps staging coordinator. Many patients will wish for further discussion; this can then take place in a more relaxed atmosphere where patients can have an hour or more to discuss the implications of diagnosis and the impending surgery with a knowledgeable and sympathetic ear. The colorectal nurse practitioner can also access a number of other key personnel such as stoma therapists to discuss temporary covering stomas or permanent stomas, so the patients' appropriate expectations are met during surgery. There is also an opportunity at these sessions to go into more depth about family history and the question of screening siblings and children if that is appropriate.

Patients who are found to have advanced disease may have alternatives to major surgery discussed with them, such as radiochemotherapy, laser, argon diathermy or local surgical procedures that may obviate the need for major resection and not alter the prognosis for that particular patient. Similarly, the appropriateness of a simple defunctioning stoma to treat patients symptomatically under these circumstances can also be discussed.

As far as consent is concerned, this should be undertaken by the operating surgeon and his team. However, it would be wrong to assume that the short discussion after admission on the day before surgery, during bowel preparation, is adequate in terms of the consent procedure. Not only do the generalized risks of surgery as far as morbidity and mortality are concerned need to be discussed with the patient, but also any specific morbidity or mortality risk that may be associated with the patient's own medical history. Many of these patients are elderly and have concomitant medical conditions that increase the risk considerably. Encouragement can also be given at this point to decrease some of the concomitant risks, e.g. stopping smoking some 4–6 weeks before an operation will significantly reduce the risk of cardiovascular complications. Similarly, those patients who have known cardiac or peripheral vascular disease have an increased risk of myocardial infarction and strokes. Despite surgeons' best efforts, there is a significant mortality rate associated with operating on patients with colon and rectal cancer, and the patient and his or her family should understand this.

Before hospital admission, the patient will be offered an opportunity to meet the nurse practitioner and discuss the reasons for surgery. The patient will be offered a clear explanation of which segment of colon the surgeon plans to remove and the impact that surgery will have on future bowel function. At this meeting, pre- and postoperative care is explained so that the patient and his or her family are aware of what to expect. Each aspect of nursing care is discussed including:

- Admission and orientation to the ward
- Preoperative bowel preparation blood tests, ECG, chest radiograph, etc.
- Physiotherapy input and the importance of postoperative exercises
- The delivery of oxygen and the monitoring of oxygen saturation in the blood
- The central infusion line and what fluids could be delivered postoperatively, e.g. clear fluids for hydration, potential blood transfusion, antibiotics, antiemetics, etc.
- The importance of monitoring the patient's vital signs
- The epidural infusion and patient control of bolus doses of pain relief
- Wound placement and dressings
- Stoma formation and potential drain sites
- Urinary catheter and the reasons for monitoring of urine output
- Antiembolic stockings and prophylaxis for deep venous thrombosis (DVT).

As each aspect of surgery is explained, the potential complications are also discussed, thereby ensuring that, when consent for surgery is obtained from the patient, it is informed consent. The patient should also be aware of the potential problems of surgery and understand that there is a 1–2% chance of a permanent stoma following any major bowel surgery. It is our experience that patients really appreciate this opportunity to discuss with the nurse practitioner the information that was given to them by the consultant. The discussion with the nurse practitioner takes place when the patient has had time to evaluate the initial information. If the nurse practitioner has built a rapport with the patient during investigations, it is helpful if he or she is present when the patient receives the diagnosis.

Much emphasis is placed on the patient's understanding of why events proceed as they do and how this knowledge allows the patients to assist in their own recovery. If a patient is aware that effective pain control leads to ease of movement, and that this in turn increases circulation and helps to prevent complications such as chest infection and DVT, that patient is less likely to suffer in silence but to be aware of the effectiveness of their pain control. Effective pain control allows the patient actively to take part in the exercises with the physiotherapist and mobilize more effectively. It is envisaged that by giving patients information before hospital admission they will be less anxious. This basic information also enables patients to ask further questions of the ward staff from an increased knowledge base. There are now multimedia computer programs available to use during these counselling sessions. It would seem appropriate to use these, depending on the capacity of the patient. As many discuss complex risks related to surgery, chemotherapy and radiotherapy, it is unlikely that these would be used in a situation without the nurse practitioner controlling the progress through the program and the information received by the patient.

In summary, the time between diagnosis and surgery or alternative therapy, in addition to staging the tumours, is a good opportunity to provide information for patients and their relatives about the surgical options and the likely outcomes and risks. In addition, there is an opportunity to talk through any family risks that may be associated with the diagnosis, and therefore give patients adequate information that allows them to come to surgery with sufficient knowledge of their disease and the proposed treatment so that they can give properly informed consent.

Staging of the cancer after surgery by the histopathologist is discussed and also an explanation given about possible postoperative treatments, i.e. chemotherapy alone or chemo-/radiotherapy. This is not discussed in great detail at this point but is mentioned to allow a channel of communication to be opened should it be needed after surgery. After discharge the patients have the support of the ward, nurse practitioner and stoma team (if appropriate). A telephone number is provided and the patient can contact the hospital with any worries or questions.

Surgical intervention

Cancers arising within the colon will require segmental resection. This is a relatively standard procedure, differing only in the segment of bowel resected.

Cancers of the right hemicolon

Cancer that affects the right hemicolon can arise anywhere from the terminal ileum to the mid-transverse colon. As discussed earlier, right-sided cancers account for 30% of colorectal cancers. Patients who present with cancers in the right side of the colon most probably suffer vague abdominal pains; obstruction is unusual in this side of the colon owing to the liquid nature of faeces. Patients may have developed anaemia; FOB testing is helpful in alerting the GP to occult bleeding from this area, but only if undertaken correctly. The patient may present with a change of bowel habit and/or unexplained weight loss and possible lethargy. As a result of the insidious nature of the onset of the disease, right-sided cancers may be more advanced at first presentation.

Diagnosis of right-sided lesions is usually made from barium enema or colonoscopy (occasionally CT). Either investigation would be ordered after initial assessment in the outpatients department. Assessment would include a full oral history, abdominal examination and a rigid or flexible sigmoidoscopy. Small bowel symptoms may be suggestive of a right-sided lesion. Occasionally, a small bowel enema will identify a lesion at the junction of the terminal ileum and the ileocaecal valve.

The removal of the right half of the colon will result in an altered bowel habit. Patients may have increased frequency and possible loose stools in the early months after surgery. This will improve over the months and by the time a patient is 6–12 months after surgery their bowel habits should have settled into a regular pattern. Patients accept that this slight increase in frequency is a small inconvenience to pay for the knowledge that the cancer has been removed. It is important that the patient is aware of the slight possibility of a temporary stoma after this surgery. Temporary ileostomy is very rarely required when surgery is performed on the right side of the colon, but stoma possibility should always be explained to the patient undergoing colorectal resection.

Right hemicolectomy

This operation is performed for cancers lying in the right half of the colon, proximal to the splenic flexure. For those cancers proximal to the hepatic flexure, a simple right hemicolectomy with an ileotransverse colon anastomosis is usually performed (Figure 6.1). For cancers in the transverse colon, an extended right hemicolectomy, taking the whole of the right and the transverse colon with an anastomosis between the ileum and the left side of the colon, is usually undertaken.

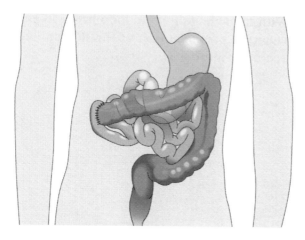

Figure 6.1 Right hemicolectomy: resection can also include the transverse colon up to the splenic flexure.

Cancers of the left hemicolon

Cancers that arise in the left half of the colon in the area, from the splenic flexure to the sigmoid colon, are removed by left hemicolectomy. Left-sided cancers account for up to 70% of colon and rectal cancers, but this also includes cancers arising in the rectum. To detect cancers in this area of the bowel, the patient will have undergone a flexible sigmoidoscopy, colonoscopy or barium enema. Patients may present with abdominal pain, change in bowel habit and/or fullness in the left side of the abdomen.

Removal of the left hemicolon will result in an increase in frequency of defecation. As with right hemicolectomy, the patient will notice an improvement over the postoperative period settling into a regular pattern by around 6-12 months after surgery. The risk of temporary ileostomy is slightly higher in left as opposed to right hemicolectomy but remains low at around 10%; this should be discussed with the patient.

Left hemicolectomy

This operation is performed for cancers in the left side of the colon, including the sigmoid colon, and can involve a left hemi-colectomy, where the left side of the colon is removed and a transverse-to-sigmoid anastomosis is undertaken. For lesions in the sigmoid colon, this area, and perhaps the upper rectum, are removed. With the splenic flexure mobilized, an anastomosis is made between the proximal part of the descending colon and the upper rectum (Figure 6.2).

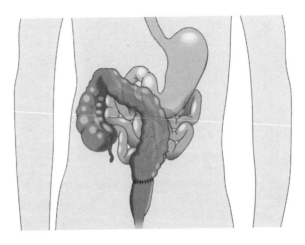

Figure 6.2 Extended left hemicolectomy.

Cancers of the rectum

Cancers of the rectum can arise from the anal verge to the rectosigmoid junction. These cancers account for up to half of the cancers that arise in the left side of the bowel. The patient may present with a sensation of tenesmus (a painful, ineffective need to empty the rectum); they may notice a change in bowel habit towards either diarrhoea or constipation. They may also notice a change in the diameter of their stool and sometimes describe explosive bowel movements. There could also be painful or painless rectal bleeding. Diagnosis of rectal cancer may be made by rigid sigmoidoscopy, flexible sigmoidoscopy, colonoscopy or barium enema.

Rectal cancer can be treated in a number of ways. High rectal cancer arising 10–15 cm from the anal verge can be treated with an anterior resection and the patient has a good chance of retaining their gastrointestinal continuity. This patient may well require a temporary ileostomy to cover the healing anastomosis, but rarely requires a permanent colostomy. Lower rectal cancers that arise between the anal verge and 8–10 cm pose a problem for the surgeon. Reconstruction of gastrointestinal continuity is preferable but it may, in some cases, be necessary to sacrifice the anal sphincters in order to achieve a surgical cure.

It has been suggested that patients with rectal cancer can benefit from preoperative radiotherapy to 'shrink' or 'down-stage' the tumour. A Swedish trial of treatment for rectal cancer has resulted in recommendations that all patients with rectal cancer, arising less than 15 cm from the anal verge, should undergo at least a short course of radiotherapy (Swedish Rectal Cancer Trial, 1997). The trial claims that a preoperative 5-day course of radiotherapy will decrease the risk of local recurrence and, providing that surgery is undertaken within 10 days, with no increased morbidity. A randomized controlled trial run by the Medical Research Council (2002) is at present under way in the UK to evaluate this treatment.

Anterior resection and abdominoperineal resection of rectum

Rectal cancers are treated by anterior resection of the rectum with a restorative anastomosis made between the left side of the colon and the remaining rectum after the resection. If the rectal cancer is close to the anal canal and it is not possible to get more than 2-cm clearance below that for the anastomosis, it is generally treated by abdominoperineal resection (APER) and permanent colostomy (Figure 6.3).

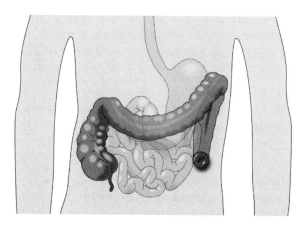

Figure 6.3 Abdominoperineal resection (APER): shows the maximum extent of bowel resection.

Total or subtotal colectomy

Patients occasionally present with synchronous lesions within the colon and the surgeon is then left with the dilemma of which resection to undertake. There is a group of patients for whom the operation of choice is a total or subtotal colectomy. It should be considered that, if a patient has already produced two lesions within the colon, there is a potential to produce more and colectomy would prevent this. For patients with ulcerative colitis or multiple adenomatous polyps, the operations of choice are total colectomy with an ileorectal anastomosis or a panproctocolectomy with an ileoanal pouch. It is not usual practice to perform panproctocolectomy with an ileoanal pouch on patients who have a cancer diagnosis, but it has occasionally been performed for multiple polyps, and when the specimen has been examined adenocarcinoma has been diagnosed. Patients undergoing subtotal colectomy with ileorectal anastomosis will need to be well motivated. They will have increased bowel movements and may defecate between four and eight times a day when their bowel has settled into a pattern. Improved control of output can be obtained by using drugs such as loperamide (Imodium) or codeine.

Postoperative follow-up

Follow-up of patients who have undergone surgery for colon or rectal cancer is routinely carried out over a 5-year period. It includes rigid sigmoidoscopy, abdominal examination, routine blood tests, chest radiographs and colonic imaging. It also requires CT or MRI of the liver for the first 2 years postoperatively. The nature of follow-up for these patients lends itself to nurse-led care. These patients are usually well and their needs are for reassurance and information. Many patients focus only on their forthcoming operation after a diagnosis of colon or rectal cancer, so it is not until after they have undergone surgery that the full impact of the diagnosis is realized. It is at this stage that further information and support are needed. The care delivered by the nurse practitioner can be designed with these patient needs in mind, thus providing the patient with a support system and reducing the workload on the consultant clinics. By following a set protocol, safe and effective, patient-oriented, follow-up care can be delivered by a nurse practitioner who has close contact with the medical team.

Prognosis

The factors that predict a good prognosis for the patient are in all cases clear radial margins, no lymph node involvement and a cancer that has not breached the bowel wall. This information is obtained from the histopathologist after examination of the resected specimen. The prognosis in colon and rectal cancer relates to the stage of the disease. Dukes' staging is generally used in the UK and Europe, and a modified form of this, called the Aster–Coller classification, is used in the USA. The international staging is the TNM (tumour, nodes, metastases) classification, as defined by Henson et al. (1994). In Dukes' A patients, the cancer is limited to the mucosa and does not invade the muscularis propria. The 5-year survival rate is between 90 and 95%. No further treatment is normally undertaken in the way of chemo-/radiotherapy for these patients, but it should be remembered that failure is usually associated with metastatic disease, so they do require continuous and adequate follow-up to assess the abdomen and liver.

In Dukes' B lesions, the cancer has bridged the muscularis propria and variably penetrated through the bowel wall and into the serosa. There are, however, no associated lymph node metastases and the 5-year survival rate is reported as between 50 and 75%. The difficulty with diagnosing Dukes' B cancer is the number of lymph nodes that are actually sampled looking for metastatic disease; if this number is low, clearly a potential Dukes' C cancer would be missed, along with the requirement for further therapy.

In Dukes' C cancer, the lymph nodes contain metastatic cancer. The reported 5-year survival rate for these patients is between 30 and 50% and the current evidence suggests that this can be improved significantly with postoperative chemotherapy.

Dukes' D cancer is a misnomer. There was no D classification in Dukes' original staging. This has, however, now been adopted for any of the above stages of colorectal cancer with evidence of metastatic spread. The prognosis is correspondingly poor with a 5-year survival rate of less than 5%.

Further treatment

Postoperative chemotherapy has already been mentioned above and evidence from American studies, and increasingly from European studies, is that patients with Dukes' C cancer will benefit with an increase in the 5-year survival period of between 5 and 15% from postoperative chemotherapy (Moertel, 1994). The chemotherapy regimens are based on 5-fluorouracil and this treatment should be undertaken in conjunction with an oncologist who has a special interest in colorectal cancer.

It has been suggested that chemotherapy may also benefit patients with Dukes' B disease but the indications are far less clear and this is the subject of ongoing debate. Although there may be a small increase in 5-year survival, there has also been the suggestion that this reflects an improvement in survival of cancers that were understaged as B, when they were really C, but lymph node metastases were not identified at pathological assessment.

Radiotherapy has little role to play in colonic cancer but it may well have a role to play in rectal cancer. Preoperative radiotherapy can be used to downstage large rectal cancers to make them operable and, in this case, a full long-course radiotherapy over 4 or 5 weeks, with or without the addition of chemotherapy at the beginning and the end, is currently the treatment of choice. As discussed earlier, in patients with operable cancer there is evidence from Swedish studies that short-course radiotherapy in the preoperative period will decrease the instance of local recurrence by anything up to 20%. In patients whose rectal cancer is incompletely excised, or where the margins are very close, there may be a rationale for offering them postoperative radiotherapy to attempt to reduce the risk of local recurrence.

Multidisciplinary care

Patients who are treated within a colorectal unit are referred for many and varied reasons. The surgery undertaken usually involves a segmental resection of some sort. The role of the nurse practitioner within the multidisciplinary team is one of patient advocate. The nurse practitioner can be a point of contact for the patient from the start of their journey through the unit to their eventual discharge after 5 years of disease-free follow-up. Close professional relationships are essential for the role to achieve its full potential, but the rewards for the practitioner and colleagues are immense. There is no doubt that colon and rectal cancer is a devastating disease for the patient and his or her family. However, effective multidisciplinary care and support delivered by a cohesive and motivated team can alleviate some of the devastating effects and allow the patient and family to resume some degree of normality in their lives.

References

Burke W, Peterson G, Lynch P, for the Cancer Genetics Studies Consortium (1997) Recommendations for follow-up care of individuals with an inherited predisposition to cancer. 1 Hereditary nonpolyposis colon cancer. Journal of the American Medical Association 1997; 277: 915–919.

Henson et al. (1994) Cited in Keighley M, Williams N (1999) Surgery of the Anus, Rectum and Colon, 2nd edn. London: Harcourt Brace & Co.

Houston RS, Murday V, Harocopos C, Williams CB, Slack J (1990) Screening and genetics counselling for relatives of patients with colorectal cancer in a family cancer clinic. British Medical Journal 301: 366–368.

Hughes MAP, Keng V, Hartley J et al. (1999) A randomised trial comparing nurses and doctors performing flexible sigmoidoscopy. Paper presented at Brighton, ASCPGBI July 2000.

Joint Advisory Group on Gastrointestinal Endoscopy (1999) Recommendations for Training in Gastrointestinal Endoscopy. JCHMT.

Medical Research Council Colorectal Cancer Working Party (2002) Randomised trial comparing pre-operative radiotherapy and selective post-operative chemoradiotherapy in rectal cancer. CR07 ongoing trial. Cambridge: MRC Cancer Trials Office.

Moertel CG (1994) Chemotherapy for colorectal cancer. New England Journal of Medicine 330: 1136–1142.

Swedish Rectal Cancer Trial (1997) Improved survival with preoperative radiotherapy in resectable rectal cancer. New England Journal of Medicine 336: 980–987.

CHAPTER 7

Nutrition and gastrointestinal cancer

DIANE PALMER AND PAMELA BARKER

Eating is fundamental and occupies a lot of our attention; concerns about nutrition are frequently in the media, with many 'alternative' diets being suggested as preventing or curing cancer. Despite this level of interest in the lay press, it is unfortunate that many health professionals tend to ignore nutrition until patients have severe symptoms.

It has been suggested that modification of diet can reduce the risk of cancer development, and that for all ages a dietary risk-reduction approach should be practised. Furthermore, at times of stress and illness the importance of adequate nutrition should not be underestimated; significant benefits can be achieved by maintaining nutritional status and weight during illness.

This chapter explores the evidence that indicates that a cancer risk-reduction diet should be advocated, which, in addition to identifying factors, may help to maintain and improve nutritional status for the person with cancer. It is not the authors' intention to consider all aspects of diet, nutrients and cancer, but rather to indicate to the nurse practitioner some simple advice and guidance, which may be passed on to patients or indeed their families and friends with confidence. The chapter has two halves: the first focuses on nutrition in relation to the prevention of cancer and the second on issues relating to nutrition in patients with cancer from diagnosis, through treatment and finally palliative care.

Associations between diet and the development of cancer

The ability of diet to influence the development of cancer has been a popular research subject for many years; however, the evidence linking diet with cancer remains difficult to evaluate, usually as a result of design limitations of the studies and the complexities of analysing such data.

Gastrointestinal (GI) cancer is thought to be related to both environmental and endogenous factors. Although there is no definite proof that diet and cancer are related, there are trends suggesting strong associations. These trends are particularly associated with diets high in saturated fats and low in vegetable and fruit consumption, in addition to the already recognized associations of genetics and smoking. The largely tenuous evidence linking diet with cancer is the result of the nature of collecting epidemiological data and problems associated with assessment of food consumption. Under- and over-reporting of food intake has occurred in many studies, although more recently large cohort world studies have attempted to standardize data recording.

It is thought that nutritional imbalance is the contributor to cancer aetiology. This includes both excess and inadequacy of nutrients. Current evidence seems to favour the association between fruit and vegetable consumption and protection against cancer (Block et al., 1992), these foods being linked to lower mortality in the cancer patient (Steinmetz and Potter, 1991a, Ziegler, 1991). A diet low in fruit and vegetables may result in inadequate levels of antioxidants, whereas a diet high in these foods should provide phytochemicals recognized to have protective effects (Cargay, 1992).

It is difficult to determine one particular factor that may contribute to the development of cancer in the GI tract. In the colon and rectum, for example, there is now evidence that high meat and low vegetable consumption may increase the risk of cancer, along with weight gain and a diet low in non-starch polysaccharides (cereals, vegetables and fruit); however, genetic make-up also plays a large part (Welfare, 1999). Studies of populations who have migrated from areas where cancer risk was low to high-risk areas have identified that migrating populations adopt the cancer rates of the new environment, probably caused by adopting the diet of the new environment (Willett, 1997).

Despite vast health promotion campaigns many people seem reluctant to alter their dietary habits. Thomas (1996) suggests that this may be caused by ambiguity, for the average person, of the exact meaning of terms such as low-fat or high-fibre diet.

This problem may be compounded by conflicting advice, because many health professionals themselves are unsure of the most up-to-date evidence.

The ease of convenience foods now available has had an impact on eating habits in the Western World. The pressures of working and bringing up a family make the option of these foods very attractive. Unfortunately, however, they often tend to be high in fat and sugar, and it is unlikely that fresh vegetables or fruit will be eaten as an accompaniment. The art of cooking has declined with the increased availability of the ready-made and 'fast foods', which will inevitably affect the next generation. This has already been seen in America where, despite the American Cancer Society (1996) health promotion initiatives, the American population is failing to adopt a diet that promotes health. The lack of adoption of healthy eating advice also coincides with an increase in tobacco smoking among teenagers.

Advice on foods known to promote health and thought to decrease associated risks of cancer should focus on a varied diet, incorporating five servings of fruit and vegetables each day. The current guidelines for healthy eating are outlined in Table 7.1. The most important factors suggested as lessening the chances of developing cancer are to avoid obesity and reduce intake of high-fat foods. Obesity is particularly associated with cancer of the uterus, gallbladder, kidney, stomach, colon and breast.

Table 7.1 General healthy eating guidelines

Eat five or more portions of fruit and/or vegetables every day
Choose most foods from plant sources
Restrict intake of fat foods, particularly from animal sources
Stay within your healthy weight range
Be at least moderately active for 30 minutes each day
Restrict alcohol intake

Healthy eating and cancer prevention

Many fruits and vegetables are now recognized as beneficial foods as a result of their high antioxidant content, which protects cell membranes against oxidative damage and may have an inhibitive effect on cancer development. Although there is currently no 'definite' evidence on the role of antioxidants and their relationship to cancer prevention, they are known to protect the body against oxygen-induced damage to tissues. There is, however, 'convincing' evidence to suggest that a high intake of fruit and vegetables decreases the risk of developing oral, oesophageal and stomach cancer, with vegetables alone showing a decrease in the risk of colorectal cancer (World Cancer Research Fund and American Institute for Cancer Research, 1997). Therefore, it appears that increasing intake of antioxidants is just as important as restricting exposure to carcinogens.

Antioxidants are found in vitamins E and C, selenium and β-carotene. Table 7.2 lists some of the rich food sources of these nutrients. It is recognized that changing a diet drastically is difficult because the types of food we eat and the way we prepare food are learnt from an early age and are often habitual. Healthy eating guidelines should concentrate on encouraging a healthy diet without taking away the enjoyment of food. Changing a diet slightly can improve one's health without too great an effect on family life. Families on low income may find it difficult to adapt to a healthier diet, the priority being to purchase food that the children will eat, rather than food that may be wasted. However, as cancer risk can be reduced by 30–40% through simple alterations to the diet (World Cancer Research Fund and American Institute for Cancer Research, 1997), the importance of changing eating behaviour should not be overlooked.

Table 7.2 Rich sources of antioxidants

Micro-nutrient	Food
Selenium	Kidney, liver, cereal, meat, diary products, sea foods
Vitamin E	Almonds, cod liver oil, peanuts, butter, margarine, fortified cereal, cream, leafy green vegetables
Vitamin C	Citrus fruits, tomatoes, potatoes, broccoli, watercress, peppers, berries
Beta-carotene	Fruit and vegetables, especially yellow and red fruits

Simple advice using non-complicated language and examples should help to avoid confusion. The message to present is that healthy eating does not need to be expensive, boring or restrictive; diet modification rather than complete change is more likely to produce lasting effects. The Health Education Council in the UK has produced guidelines in an effort to simplify nutritional recommendations. Examples of advice similar to that offered by the Health Education Authority (1994) are illustrated in Table 7.3.

Table 7.3 Healthy food options

Breads/cereals, pasta, rice and potato
These should form one-third of the total daily diet. Ideally high-fibre bread and brown rice and pasta should be selected. Boiled potatoes will be healthier than fried although additions of butter and margarine will influence the value of the diet

Fruit and vegetables
As a minimum, five portions daily should be the aim

Milk and dairy products
This should make up one-sixth of the total daily diet, with lower-fat alternatives being selected

Meat, poultry, fish
Choose lower-fat alternatives and eat without the skin. Avoid adding additional fat when cooking. White meat and fish are generally lower in fat than dark meat. Pulses are a good low-fat alternative to meat

Cakes, sweets, biscuits and snacks foods
These should contribute to only one-twelfth of the total daily dietary intake, and include crisps, pastry, carbonated drinks, oils, dressings and cream

---

Nutrition and GI tract cancers

Head and neck cancer

Smoking and alcohol are the two major risk factors associated with oral cancers, usually affecting the oral cavity, larynx and oesophagus; the risk increases when both factors are present. Certain vitamins and minerals are suppressed with smoking and alcohol consumption, in particular vitamin B_{12}, folate and retinoids. It is thought that in oral and pharyngeal cancer the lower consumption of vegetables and fruit with a high consumption of salt-preserved meat or fish may be a contributory factor (Winn, 1995), although when compared with smoking and alcohol the effects of diet are modest (Department of Health, 1998).

There is convincing evidence that a diet high in fruit and vegetables decreases the risk of pharyngeal, mouth and laryngeal cancers, probably as a result of the protective mechanism of the fruit and vegetables, with the intake of yellow and green vegetables showing promising results (Gridley et al., 1992).

Oesophageal cancer

There is a distinct geographical feature to this cancer with a higher risk associated with poorer countries and those areas with a compromised diet, such as north central China, central Asia and northern Iran. Mineral deficiency may be attributable to the development of oesophageal cancer along with hot drinks, pickled foods and mouldy foods containing aflatoxin (World Cancer Research Fund and American Institute for Cancer Research, 1997). Aflatoxin has been found to be carcinogenic in animal studies and is thought to be a cause of primary cancer in humans. It binds to cellular DNA and is associated with mutation of the p53 tumour-suppressor gene, which is important in the development of some human cancers (Hsu et al., 1991).

The beneficial effects of vitamin C have been associated with a reduction in oesophageal cancer. A correlation between high serum levels of ascorbic acid and a decreased risk of mortality from oesophageal cancer has been identified from epidemiological studies (Brown et al., 1988; Chen et al., 1992).

Gastric cancer

An increased risk of gastric cancer has been associated with a preference for salty and pickled foods (Coggon et al., 1989), which induce gastritis leading to damage of the protective mucosal layer of the stomach.

It is generally thought that a diet high in fruit and vegetables will reduce the risk of gastric cancer. Refrigeration of foods and the availability of different types of fruit and vegetables all year round have had an impact on reducing the incidence of gastric cancers throughout the world. This may result, in part, from the prolonged preservation of fruit and vegetables provided by freezing, which has caused a reduction in mould growth and less requirement for food to be salted for preservation.

Colorectal cancer

There is substantial evidence from both population and laboratory studies to suggest that diets high in fat may increase the risk of colon cancer and diets high in fibre may reduce the risk. Recent investigations have identified that people with a family history of colon cancer may be at higher risk from an adverse diet (Slattery and Potter, 1997).

Heavily burnt meats, particularly red meats, are thought to be linked to cancer development because of the production of heterocyclic amines, which are pro-carcinogens (Welfare, 1999). Studies have identified consumers of fried meat with a heavily browned surface being at a higher risk of colorectal cancer (Gerhardsson de Verdier et al., 1991; Probst-Hensch et al., 1997).

In countries where a high-fibre diet is consumed, such as African populations, there is a low incidence of colon cancer (Burkitt, 1969). It is thought that the fermenting process of some soluble fibre may have a protective effect against carcinogens on the colonic mucosa (Thomas, 1996). Dietary fish oils are also thought to play a part in protecting against colon cancer (Bartram et al., 1993), although more evidence is needed to substantiate this claim.

There is convincing evidence that a diet rich in vegetables has protective effects against the development of cancers in the colon and rectum. Vegetables contain micronutrients and bioactive compounds such as flavonoids, which are thought to have anti-carcinogenic properties (Steinmetz and Potter, 1991b). However, they are also a rich source of fibre, along with the non-digestible fructo-oligosaccharides associated with selective promotion of beneficial bacteria such as *Lactobacillus* and *Bifidobacterium* species (Gibson and Roberfroid, 1996). In particular, cruciferous vegetables such as broccoli and cabbage have been associated with a reduced risk of colorectal cancer (Benito et al., 1990).

Liver and pancreatic cancer

The incidence of pancreatic cancer differs significantly in population studies with the highest rates in western Europe and the USA, whereas Asia and Africa have lower rates. Diets high in fat and low in vegetable consumption may contribute to development of pancreatic cancer, whereas vitamin C and fibre may have a protective role. There is also a possible association between cancer of the liver and pancreas and a high intake of coffee combined with a low intake of fruit (World Cancer Research Fund and American Institute for Cancer Research, 1997).

General advice

As previously mentioned, evidence of associations between diet and cancer are not always clear and to date are largely formulated from retrospective population studies. The reliability of this method of data collection is known to be problematic and as such definitive conclusions and recommendations are difficult to validate. We therefore have opted to report food links with cancer that consistently recur in many studies, where the evidence relies on a variety of methods of reporting. However, it is likely that controversy and doubt will remain for some time to come. We therefore suggest that dietary advice should focus on the following:

- The diet should be balanced, incorporating a variety of foods primarily of plant origin such as fresh fruit, vegetables and pulses.
- If red meat is to be eaten, it should be restricted to a quantity of no more than 80 g (3 oz) each day; however, poultry or fish is a preferable option.
- Although alcohol consumption is not recommended, if it is consumed it should be restricted to less than two units each day for men and one for women.
- Dramatic weight fluctuation should be avoided, with reliance on regular exercise rather than reduction diets being selected when weight control is a problem.
- Smoking cessation is strongly advocated.

Diet and the cancer patient

Treatment, therapies and associated side effects of cancer may all contribute to nutritional depletion. The effect may be obvious such as malabsorption of nutrients after gastrectomy, or indirect such as increased metabolic demands, e.g. as a result of infection. The nurse's role in assessing and addressing nutritional status should be a priority in patient care (Whitman, 2000).

Tumour effects

Nutritional problems may be experienced as a result of the direct effect of the tumour. An enlarging tumour may impair GI tract function, leading to nausea, vomiting, reduced transit times, malabsorption and possibly obstruction. Early satiety may be associated with ascites, which can also lead to fluid and electrolyte disturbances. Pain from the tumour site may diminish the desire to eat, whereas confusion caused by pressure from central nervous system tumours may restrict cognitive function to the extent that a person forgets to eat. Decreased oral intake may result in nitrogen imbalance and a decrease in fat mobilization may occur (De Wys, 1980), with metabolic alterations producing glucose intolerance.

Weight loss and its effects

De Wys and colleagues (1980) found that patients who presented with weight loss at the time of initial diagnosis had significantly less survival time after therapy than patients who presented with no weight loss. This suggests that significant weight loss is associated with poor prognosis. It affects about 80% of patients with cancer of the stomach and 54% of patients with cancer of the colon at the time of diagnosis (De Wys et al., 1980). Early recognition of weight loss is required for successful prevention of further deterioration of body composition and performance.

Weight loss may be caused by complications of the tumour, e.g. abdominal distension or obstruction. However, it may be attributed to the treatment; mouth ulcers and taste alterations inhibit the desire to eat, whereas anxiety may induce early satiety. The loss of 10% or more of body weight in the previous 3 months correlates with protein–energy malnutrition. However, the absence of weight loss may not necessarily represent normal nutritional status. Indeed, weight gain may indicate fluid retention, representing albumin and function energy loss and muscle wasting. Causes of reduced nutritional status are listed in Table 7.4.

Table 7.4 Causes of reduced nutritional status

Loss of appetite
Severe weight loss
Hypoproteinaemia
Oedema
Muscle atrophy
Fatigue
Malaise

Cancer cachexia and anorexia

Cachexia is a clinical wasting syndrome often associated with anorexia, although not exclusively. It may occur in people who are eating sufficient protein and calories, but have diminished absorption. Symptoms of cancer cachexia are listed in Table 7.5. Often unrelated to food intake or tumour site, it is characterized by weakness accompanied by severe loss of weight, muscle and fat. Patients experience cachexia with no obvious cause for their weight loss, which is recognized as a metabolic syndrome probably resulting from an endogenous response of the host. Cytokines and hormones released by the tumour and host cells are thought to be mediators of the cachexia.

Table 7.5 Symptoms of cancer cachexia

Altered taste and smell
Increased energy expenditure
Anxiety
Depression
Nausea and vomiting
Early satiety
Diarrhoea
Obstruction

Anorexia is simply the loss of appetite or desire to eat, and affects 15–25% of people with cancer at the time of diagnosis (Langstein and Norton, 1991). It may be caused by the pathophysiology of the disease or from anxiety resulting from the disease status. Patients often complain of loss of appetite in addition to modification of taste and decrease of smell, all resulting in decreased food intake. Depression and conditioned food aversion may contribute to mechanisms of anorexia (Bernstein and Bernstein, 1981). Metabolites such as oligonucleotides and peptides produced by the cancer cells may alter taste sensations. Other problems caused by emotional distress, leading to eating disturbances, are nausea, abdominal discomfort, constipation and diarrhoea.

Strong food odours can induce anorexia, so it may be advisable to encourage cold foods, which are less pungent, or the patient should not be involved with food preparation. Strong aromas can be reduced by boiling food in bags, serving on cold plates or, when the weather permits, cooking food outside. If a metallic taste is present when eating, this may be reduced by the provision of plastic utensils.

Psychosocial issues

Eating is a social activity enjoyed by many. When the appetite is lost, this activity obviously no longer holds the same appeal. Instantly a family and social activity are relinquished, and the person with anorexia or food aversion becomes socially isolated. When an unpleasant symptom has been encountered after eating a specific food, aversions are soon acquired, contributing to reduced desire to eat (Bernstein, 1982). Large helpings can be overpowering; small helpings on small plates are easier to manage, and a little more can always be added if the appetite allows. Cultural eating preferences and altered appetite may severely restrict the type and quantity of food eaten. It is also important to remember that other social and psychosocial factors such as living alone and the lack of energy to prepare food can contribute to a reduced food intake. Mild exercise such as walking should be encouraged where possible because it is also associated with a reduction in nausea and vomiting and increased desire to eat (Ottery, 1994).

Lethargy and apathy are often experienced by the cancer victim, with motivation being affected by under-nutrition (Mays, 1995). It has been suggested that protein–energy malnutrition-associated apathy and depression may be caused by low tyrosine, affecting brain neurotransmitters (Antener et al., 1981). Studies on healthy adults have identified that, when weight loss exceeds 10% of normal body weight, mental performance begins to be affected, with a disruption to cognitive function manifesting as lethargy, helplessness, hypochondria and memory loss (Shippee et al., 1994; Mays, 1995).

Nutritional assessment and screening

Malnutrition is affected by tumour type, stage of disease and anti-neoplastic therapy. This means that at various stages during the illness the nutritional status of the patient may be compromised. Individual nutritional assessment of the patient is vital to the overall management. Assessment may include: the healthy individual requiring advice about decreasing their risk of developing cancer; the newly diagnosed patient who has no nutritional limitations and is not compromised but may be at risk during therapy; the patient in the midst of treatment; and the person who is post-treatment.

Screening

The important role of nurses in nutrition screening and assessment appears to have been eroded or neglected (Millar and Torrance, 1991). Nurse practitioners are not likely to provide education or counselling about diet and cancer (Tessaro et al., 1996), generally because they no longer recognize that advice on eating and diet is within their role. As the nurse is often one of the first points of patient contact, the problem of detection of the 'at-risk patient' and referral to the dietitian remains. The way forward must be for more effective collaboration between nursing staff and the registered dietitian, along with recognition that nurses and doctors have an important role to play in assessment of the elementary indicators of protein–energy malnutrition.

The recommendations of the British Association for Parenteral and Enteral Nutrition (BAPEN) for initial screening require the following simple steps:

- Weigh the patient
- Ascertain normal weight and height
- Determine recent weight loss
- Detail current appetite and compare with usual appetite.

These recommendations are simple enough to follow and should be sufficient to determine if there is a problem requiring more detailed assessment. Other more detailed screening tools are based on weight loss, height, dietary history, symptoms and fluid status. Depending on responses, patients are categorized according to risk. As with any screening tool, it can be effective only if the nurse completing it implements the required action and evaluates it regularly. Although validation of nutritional screening tools has been scanty and inconclusive (Lyne and Prowse, 1999), their benefit in terms of referrals to dietitians has been identified (Robshaw and Marbrow, 1995). It could, however, be argued that screening tools could be discarded in favour of clinical judgement and reasoning, if nurses had appropriate skills and motivation to detect the 'at-risk' and malnourished patient.

Assessment

Standardized criteria for assessing nutritional risk, such as the Subjective Global Assessment (SGA), require slightly more detail considering weight, weight history, dietary intake and normal intake, GI symptoms for the previous 2 weeks and performance status (Detsky et al., 1987). This assessment should, therefore, be carried out by someone with knowledge about determining adequate nutritional intake, ideally the dietitian or nutritionist.

Assessing food intake is difficult as a result of inconsistencies in reporting of portion size and inaccuracies of memory function during illness. The documentation of food intake relies on a variety of methods, with accurate measures of diet being hard to find. Some methods require all food and fluids to be weighed and measured, and some require a nutritionist to observe and document all intake consumed; these methods are costly and time-consuming, and so are usually used only in small controlled studies.

The '24-hour recall' method requires the patient to document or recall, when assessed, all food consumed during the previous 24 hours. This method requires minimal effort from the patient and is useful in clinical practice where time is limited. However, although accurate and simple, this method of dietary assessment does not take into account day-to-day variability (Willett, 1997). The gold standard for food assessment was until recently to weigh portions; however, unstructured recall consisting of a blank sheet of paper with written examples on the back has compared well with results from weighed records (Bingham et al., 1994). Unfortunately, once again, this method will not assess habitual diet, although it will give a reasonable assessment if repeated at intervals. Dietary assessment methods to improve techniques of data collection have been explored (Wynder et al., 1997), with the recording of a simple diary sheet for 24 hours having been identified as one of the most effective ways to assess food intake and deficit. Media reports of adverse effects with high-fat diets or poorly balanced nutritional intake may, however, restrict an honest record of consumed food. Furthermore, it should also be remembered that self-reporting is known to contain inaccuracies, particularly in elderly people as a result of reduction in short-term memory function (Sawaya et al., 1996).

Adding extra nourishment to foods

Each cancer patient will have individual protein and calorie requirements depending on their nutritional status and deficits. When the appetite is poor, the content of the food eaten is paramount, so calorie-loaded snacks should be encouraged at regular intervals. Small frequent snacks may be better tolerated than the traditional three meals per day. Extra nourishment can be provided from full-fat milk, butter should be encouraged rather than low-fat spread, and cream may be added to soups and casseroles. If not contraindicated, a glass of sherry, wine or beer may provide extra pleasure as well as stimulating the appetite.

Nutrition during cancer treatment

Nutritional support does not alter the outcome of the cancer, but may contribute towards an improved feeling of well-being. Before initiation of nutritional support, the requirements of the patient should be carefully considered. Consultation among the family, the competent patient and the healthcare team should ensure that everyone is aware of the goals of the support.

Inflammation of the large bowel, e.g. during radiotherapy to the pelvis, may benefit from a period of low-residue or elemental diet, which is totally absorbed in the proximal small intestine. A low-fat elemental diet does not stimulate pancreatic, biliary or gastrointestinal secretions, and so can be beneficial in symptom management; however, despite flavourings, the taste can be unpleasant so it is often administered via a tube.

When the gut is functioning, but intake via the oral route is inadequate, or not possible, enteral tube feeding for nutritional support is to be preferred. If a nasogastric feed is to be given it should be small bore (gauge Ch 8–10 or French 8–10) soft tube. This method of feeding is not without complications, particularly regurgitation leading to aspiration and tube dislodgement, not to mention the discomfort caused by the tube itself. Gastrostomy or jejunostomy tube feeding is often used for long duration support, and may be administered as intermittent, bolus or 12-hourly. Although they require a more invasive technique for insertion and are associated with complications (Botterill et al., 1998), these tubes are often preferred because they are not as uncomfortable or embarrassing as having a tube in the nose. In oesophageal cancer, dysphagia, anorexia, mucositis and vomiting can all lead to malnutrition. Nutritional support via a tube in those patients receiving chemo- and radiotherapy is well tolerated and prevents further nutritional deterioration (Bozzetti et al., 1998).

Parenteral nutrition (PN) may be considered when gut function is inadequate; however, extreme care is required. Complications of PN may be mechanical, metabolic or infectious, e.g. pneumothorax, electrolyte disturbances and line sepsis. However, these complications can be significantly reduced when administration of the PN is supervised by the multidisciplinary nutrition team (Lennard-Jones, 1992).

The use of preoperative PN should be reserved for the very malnourished patient with a preoperative weight loss of 15% and serum albumin less than 2.8 mg/dl (Veterans Affairs Total Parenteral Nutrition Cooperative Study Group, 1991). It is a successful method of support for patients who develop enterocutaneous fistulas after major GI surgery, and is of benefit to optimize nutrition for the patient with acute radiation and chemotherapy enteritis.

Surgery

Poor nutritional status will decrease resilience to surgery, radiation and chemotherapy, both physically and psychologically. Often it can be the surgical procedure itself that causes the nutritional inadequacies.

Difficulty in eating, swallowing and chewing may be experienced after head and neck surgery, and in some cases the ability to taste and smell may be lost. Some people may not be able to eat in the conventional manner and will in severe cases have to rely on tube feeding. Malnutrition induced by poor diet and eating difficulties is associated with depression in this group of patients (Westin et al., 1988). However, early and constant enteral nutrition (EN) can stabilize the nutritional state and quality of life of patients with tumours of the head and neck, particularly during radiotherapy (Senft et al., 1993).

Oesophageal surgery may result in gastric stasis and fat malabsorption as a result of vagal sectioning. After surgical treatment for cancer of the oesophagus, nutritional status is usually maintained with tube feeding (EN or PN) until the integrity of the anastomosis has been confirmed. Once oral nutrition has recommenced, meals should be small and frequent. In cases of advanced cancer, when surgery is contraindicated, a prosthetic tube (Celestin or Atkinson) may be inserted to maintain swallowing. As the diameter of the tube is fairly small, meals should be soft or liquidized. After eating, a fizzy drink should be encouraged to help to clean the tube and prevent blockage.

Gastric surgery is often associated with early satiety, malabsorption and dumping syndrome, in addition to iron, vitamin B_{12} and folate deficiencies. Although pancreatic surgery may cause vitamin and mineral deficiencies, the body adapts well to small bowel resection unless more than 70% is removed, when absorption of nutrients may become a problem.

When large bowel resection results in the creation of a stoma for the elimination of waste products, modification to the diet may be required. General guidelines should advise avoiding food found to produce excessive discomfort, although a well-balanced diet should be the overall aim. An increase in fluid intake will be necessary as more fluid is lost in the stools of people with an ileostomy, and fluid is essential to help prevent constipation for people who have a colostomy. Irregular eating patterns and fizzy drinks exacerbate flatus; some foods may produce diarrhoea and these can be avoided once they are identified as problematic. One of the main problems for people coming to terms with a stoma is learning which foods are likely to cause embarrassing odour, although the odour can be reduced by eating natural yoghurt or parsley. For the patient trying to manage a new and active stoma, reducing oral intake will reduce stoma output; however, this is not a sensible or recommended solution for a patient who is already at risk of protein–energy malnutrition after surgery.

Chemotherapy

Maintenance of nutritional status for cancer therapy patients seems to have beneficial effects on oncological therapy (Ose et al., 1998); however, the effects of chemotherapy can often result in symptoms that reduce the desire to eat.

Oral mucositis, caused by the toxicity from some chemotherapy regimens, often results in treatment delays, under-nutrition and dose reductions, although it may be possible to identify factors that predispose to development of this condition (Wilkes, 1998). Depending on the chemotherapy regimen, other side effects such as oesophagitis, malabsorption and taste alterations may occur, which all severely affect the ability to maintain adequate nutritional status. The host protein metabolism can be improved without tumour enhancement during chemotherapy, by glutamine supplementation, while a methionine-free intravenous acid solution has been shown to increase the effect of 5-fluorouracil (Katsuramaki et al., 1998). The adverse effects of cisplatin and other cytostatic drugs can be reduced by antioxidants, although it is possible that the antioxidants themselves may be consumed by the oxidative stress of the chemotherapy (Weijl et al., 1998). The role of antioxidants needs to be further explored; however, the need for a diet enriched with antioxidants in the form of fresh fruit and vegetables seems to make common sense.

Radiotherapy

Radiotherapy to the stomach and oesophagus, particularly 2–3 weeks after the start of treatment, often leads to nausea, vomiting and dyspepsia. Oesophageal mucositis can lead to dysphagia, whereas radiation-induced gastritis can cause obstruction and perforation. Patients experiencing these symptoms should be supported with a prescription for antiemetics. Antacids, antispasmodics and bland diet can all help to reduce the symptoms of dyspepsia. Small and large bowel irradiation can result in temporary irritation, producing loose stools or diarrhoea. Radiation-induced diarrhoea caused by decreased fat absorption may respond to cholestyramine, which works by binding the bile acids before they pass through the colon.

Symptom management

Therapy-related nausea and vomiting is one of the main causes of anorexia. Nausea and vomiting may be caused by chemotherapy, medications such as morphine, gastrointestinal surgery, radiotherapy, tumour invasion of the gastrointestinal tract, dumping syndrome or therapy-induced diarrhoea. Taste alterations may be the result of decreased sensitivity of the taste buds, drug interactions and nutritional deficiencies. The micronutrient zinc is important because deficiency results in taste alteration (Prasad et al., 1988); it is also an important requirement for wound healing.

Strategies to improve taste in addition to zinc supplements could include adding tarty flavourings to foods, e.g. lemon juice and vinegar. Foods that are cold, or at room temperature, often provide stronger taste than hot foods. Sometimes patients benefit from altering sweetness of foods, either reducing or increasing the levels. To mask taste that is bitter, strong seasonings or the addition of wine or beer while cooking is useful.

The desire to eat is often inhibited simply because of a dry mouth, poor mouth care or bad breath. Halitosis may be caused by poor dentition and oral care, or necrosis and sepsis of the mouth, pharynx and nose. Smoking is known to exacerbate bad breath and, indeed, gastric stagnation associated with gastric outlet obstruction. These symptoms can be reduced by a regular mouth-cleansing regimen; in addition oral candidiasis occurs commonly in the compromised patient and should always be treated. Stomatitis and xerostomia lead to decreased nutrient intake. When saliva is sparse and the mouth is dry, stimulants such as ice cubes, boiled sweets and chewing gum are useful, in addition to artificial saliva.

Alternative therapies

Dietary treatments often appear attractive to cancer patients when conventional methods are not successful. Essentially, marketing techniques, often aimed at the desperate and vulnerable, promote 'natural remedies', which are not supported by sound scientific evidence. Sensible dietary advice should be discussed with the hospital dietitian for those who are concerned about their diet, because exclusion diets may lead to weakness and weight loss.

Special diets such as those advocated by the Bristol Cancer Help Centre and Dr Max Gerson (1978) work on the principle of detoxification and require considerable effort from the patient. Indeed, there is currently no clinical evidence to support the anti-cancer effects of these diets, and strict adherence has been associated in some instances with nutrient deficiency. Arguably, however, some patients report benefit from diet therapies, although this is thought to be the result of the feeling of gaining personal control over their cancer treatment rather than the diet itself.

Palliative care

When in a palliative care situation it should be the needs of the patient, not the demands of the anxious family, that should determine whether nutritional support is appropriate. When the prognosis is poor, eating should be as pleasurable as possible without restrictions. Commercially available supplements may support food intake.

Corticosteriods provide improvement in appetite and general well-being with between 40% and 80% of patients responding to these medications (Bruera et al., 1985); however, side effects have to be considered against any positive effects of weight increase. Progestational agents, such as megestrol acetate, have been shown to support appetite stimulation and gain in body fat and mass cells (Loprinzi et al., 1990); however, in comparison to steroids it is an expensive drug and effective dosages are still being evaluated.

Conclusion

Early detection of anorexia and under-nutrition is required to prevent cachexia. The importance of diet and nutrients should not be overlooked, particularly when the GI tract is involved. When the patient is receiving treatment, alternative approaches to maintenance of nutritional status may be required and the nurse should regularly assess and evaluate food intake. Strategies to enhance the flavour of food and stimulate appetite should be considered as a regular care plan. Where cachexia cannot be prevented, anorexia can be palliated.

For patients expected to make a total recovery, the opportunity for 'healthy eating' dietary advice should not be overlooked. Evidence of the additional benefit of fruit and vegetables to the diet, particularly to the immune system, should be promoted. Diet is an important factor in the aetiology of cancer, so the healthcare professional should be aware of dietary changes to be advocated. A preventive approach, with a varied diet rich in fruit, vegetables, cereals and grains, can help in cancer risk reduction, although sensitivity, understanding and reinforced support will be required from the nurse when dietary modification is recommended.

References

American Cancer Society (1996) Advisory committee on diet, nutrition and cancer prevention. Journal of the American Cancer Society 46: 325–341.

Antener I, Tonney G, Verwilghen AM, Mauron J (1981) Biochemical study of malnutrition: Part IV. Determination of amino acids in the serum, erythrocytes, urine and stool ultrafiltrates. International Journal of Vitamins and Nutrients 51: 64–78.

Bartram HP, Gostner A, Scheppach W et al. (1993) Effects of fish oil on rectal cell proliferation, mucosal fatty acids and prostaglandin E2 release in healthy subjects. Gastroenterology 105: 1317–1322.

Benito E, Obrador A, Stiggelbout A et al. (1990) A population based case–control study of colo-rectal cancer in Majorca I Dietary Factors. International Journal of Cancer 45: 69–75.

Bernstein IL (1982) Physiological and psychological mechanisms of cancer anorexia. Cancer Research 42(suppl 2): 715s–720s.

Bernstein IL, Bernstein ID (1981) Learned food aversions and cancer anorexia. Cancer Treatment Reports 65(suppl 5): 43–47.

Bingham SA, Gill C, Welch A et al. (1994) Comparison of dietary assessment methods in nutritional epidemiology: weighed records v. 24 h recalls, food-frequency questionnaires and estimated-diet records. British Journal of Nutrition 72: 619–643.

Block G, Patterson B, Sunbar A (1992) Fruit, vegetables and cancer prevention: a review of the epidemiological evidence. Nutrition and Cancer 18: 1–29.

Botterill I, Miller G, Dexter S, Martin I (1998) Lesson of the week: deaths after delayed recognition of percutaneous endoscopic gastrostomy tube migration. British Medical Journal 317: 524–525.

Bozzetti F, Cozzaglio L, Gavazzi C et al. (1998) Nutritional support in patients with cancer of the oesophagus: impact on nutritional status, patient compliance to therapy, and survival. Tumori 84: 681–686.

Brown LM, Blot WJ, Schuman SH (1988) Environmental factors and high risk of oesophageal cancers among men in coastal Carolina. Journal of the National Cancer Institute 80: 1620–1625.

Bruera E, Roca E, Cedaro L et al. (1985) Action of oral methylprednisolone in terminal cancer patients: a prospective randomised double-blind study. Cancer Treatments Reports 69: 751–754.

Burkitt DP (1969) Related disease, related cause? Lancet ii: 1229–1231.

Cargay AB (1992) Cancer-preventative foods and ingredients. Food Technology 46: 4:65–68.

Chen J, Geissler C, Perpia B et al. (1992) Antioxidant status and cancer mortality in China. International Journal of Epidemiology 22: 625–635.

Coggon D, Barker DJP, Cole RB, Nelson M (1989) Stomach cancer and food storage. Journal of the National Cancer Institute 81: 1178–1182.

De Wys WD (1980) Nutritional care of the cancer patient. Journal of the American Medical Association 244: 374–376.

De Wys WD, Begg D, Lavin PT et al. (1980) Prognostic effect of weight loss prior to chemotherapy in cancer patients. American Journal of Medicine 69: 491.

Department of Health (1998) Nutritional Aspects of the Development of Cancer. Report of the Working Group on Diet and Cancer of the Committee on Medical Aspects of Food and Nutrition Policy. Norwich: HMSO.

Detsky AS, McLaugghlin JR, Baker JP et al. (1987) What is subjective global assessment of nutritional status? Journal of Parenteral and Enteral Nutrition 11: 8–13.

Gerhardsson de Verdier M, Hagman U, Peters RK et al. (1991) Meat, cooking methods and colorectal cancer: a case-referent study in Stockholm. International Journal of Cancer 49: 520–525.

Gerson M (1978) The cure of advanced cancer by diet therapy: a summary of 30 years of clinical experimentation. Physiological Chemistry and Physics 10: 449–464.

Gibson GR, Roberfroid MB (1996) Dietary modulation of the human colonic microbiota: introducing the concept of probiotics. Journal of Nutrition 125: 1401–1412.

Gridley G, McLaughlin JK, Block G et al. (1992) Vitamin supplement use and reduced risk of oral and pharyngeal cancer. American Journal of Epidemiology 1135: 1083–1092.

Health Education Authority (1994) The Balance of Good health. Introducing the National Food Guide. London: HEA.

Hsu IC, Metcalf RA, Sun T et al. (1991) Mutational hotspot in the p53 gene in human hepatocellular carcinomas. Nature 350: 427–428.

Katsuramaki T, Hirata K, Isobe M (1998) Nutrition and cancer patients [Review]. Journal of Japan Surgical Society 99: 187–192.

Langstein HN, Norton JA (1991) Mechanisms of cancer cachexia. Hematology/Oncology Clinics of North America 5: 103–123.

Lennard-Jones JE (1992) A Positive Approach to Nutrition as Treatment. Report of a Working Party. London: King's Fund Centre.

Loprinzi CL, Ellison NM, Schaid DJ et al. (1990) Controlled trial of megestrol acetate for the treatment of cancer anorexia and cachexia. Journal of the National Cancer Institute 82: 1127-1132.

Lyne PA, Prowse MA (1999) Methodological issues in the development and use of instruments to assess patient nutritional status or the level of risk of nutritional compromise. Journal of Advanced Nursing 30: 835-842.

Mays MZ (1995) Impact of underconsumption on cognitive performance. In: Marriott BM (ed.), Not Eating Enough: Overcoming underconsumption of military operational rations. Washington DC: National Academy Press, pp. 285-302.

Millar B, Torrance C (1991) Nutritional assessment. Surgical Nurse 4(5): 21-25.

Ose T, Blaker B, Kvaloy S et al. (1998) The importance of nutrition for cancer patients [Review]. Tidsskrift for Den Norske Laegeforening 118: 3466-3470.

Ottery FD (1994) Cancer cachexia: prevention, early diagnosis, and management. Cancer Practice 2(2): 123-131.

Prasad AS, Meftah S, Abdallah J (1988) Serum thymulin in human zinc deficiency. Journal of Clinical Investigation 82: 1202-1210.

Probst-Hensch NM, Sinha R, Longnecker MP et al. (1997) Meat preparation and colorectal adenomas in a large sigmoidoscopy-based case-control study in California (United States). Cancer Causes and Control 8: 175-183.

Robshaw V, Marbrow S (1995) Raising awareness of patient's nutritional state. Professional Nurse 11(1): 41-42.

Sawaya AL, Tucker K, Tsay R et al. (1996) Evaluation of four methods for determining energy intake in young and older women: comparison with doubly labelled water measurements of total energy expenditure. American Journal of Clinical Nutrition 63: 491-499.

Senft M, Fietau R, Iro H et al. (1993) The influence of supportive nutritional therapy via percutaneous endoscopically guided gastrostomy on the quality of life of cancer patients. Supportive Care in Cancer 1: 272-275.

Shippee R, Friedl K, Kramer T et al. (1994) Nutritional and Immunological Assessment of Ranger Students with Increased Caloric Intake. Natick, MA: US Army Research Institute of Environmental Medicine Technical Report T95-5.

Slattery ML, Potter JD (1997) Dietary fats and colon cancer: assessment of risk associated with specific fatty acids. International Journal of Cancer 73: 670-677.

Steinmetz K, Potter J (1991a) Vegetables, fruit and cancer epidemiology. Cancer Causes and Control 2(suppl): 325-357.

Steinmetz K, Potter J (1991b) Vegetables, fruit and cancer II mechanisms. Cancer Causes and Control 2(suppl): 427-442.

Tessaro IA, Herman CJ, Shaw JE, Giese EA (1996) Cancer prevention knowledge, attitudes and clinical practice of nurse practitioners in local public health departments in North Carolina. Cancer Nursing 19: 269-274.

Thomas B (1996) Nutrition in Primary Care. A handbook for health professionals. Oxford: Blackwell Science.

Veterans Affairs Total Parenteral Nutrition Cooperative Study Group (1991) Perioperative total parenteral nutrition in surgical patients. New England Journal of Medicine 325: 525.

Weijl NI, Hopman GD, Wipkink-Bakker A et al. (1998) Cisplatin combination chemotherapy induces a fall in plasma antioxidants of cancer patients. Annals of Oncology 9: 1331-1337.

Welfare M (1999) Dietary factors in colorectal cancer. International Journal of Gastroenterolgy April: 5-7.

Westin T, Jansson A, Zenckert C et al. (1988) Mental depression is associated with malnutrition in patients with head and neck cancer. Archives of Otolaryngology, Head and Neck Surgery 114: 1449-1453.

Whitman MM (2000) The starving patient: supportive care for people with cancer. Clinical Journal of Oncology Nursing 4(3): 121-125.

Wilkes JD (1998) Prevention and treatment of oral mucositis following cancer chemotherapy [Review]. Seminars in Oncology 25: 538-551.

Willett W (1997) Nutritional epidemiology: issues and challenges. International Journal of Epidemiology 16: 312-317.

Winn D (1995) Diet and nutrition in the etiology of oral cancer. American Journal of Clinical Nutrition 61: 437s-445s.

World Cancer Research Fund and American Institute for Cancer Research (1997) Food, Nutrition and the Prevention of Cancer: A global perspective. Washington, DC: American Institute for Cancer Research.

Wynder EL, Cohen LA, Winters BL (1997) The challenges of assessing fat intake in cancer research investigations [Review]. Journal of the American Dietetic Association 97(7 suppl): S5-S8.

Zeigler RG (1991) Vegetables, fruits and carotenoids and the risk of cancer. American Journal of Clinical Nutrition 53(suppl): 251-259.

CHAPTER 8

Care of the patient receiving radiotherapy

DAVINA POROCK

Radiotherapy is an unfamiliar medical treatment for most people and it is common for patients to have misconceptions about the nature of the treatment. In fact radiotherapy is used for about 60% of patients with cancer at some stage of their illness (Hilderley, 1997a; Perez and Brady, 1997). Given that one in three people in Western countries will receive a diagnosis of cancer during their lifetime (Calman and Hine, 1995; American Cancer Society, 1996), these figures mean that around 17% of all people in Western countries will undergo radiotherapy at some time in their life.

Radiotherapy is the oldest non-surgical cancer treatment and is used alone and in combination with surgery and chemotherapy in order to cure or control cancers or palliate cancer symptoms. The purpose of this chapter is to introduce the principles of radiotherapy and apply these principles to the management of radiation reactions (side effects), with particular emphasis on the reactions occurring as a result of treatment of gastrointestinal cancers. The chapter begins with an introduction to radiotherapy and radiobiology and the principles of care. This is followed by a detailed look at the effects and management of the skin and then the mucosa of the gastrointestinal tract from the oral to the colorectal mucosa and incorporating the accessory organs.

What is radiotherapy?

A brief history

Radiotherapy is a conventional anticancer treatment using ionizing radiation from either a radioactive isotope (brachytherapy) or from a megavoltage (high dose) X-ray machine called a linear accelerator (teletherapy) to eradicate tumour cells. The science and therapeutic use of ionizing radiation have developed over the past century since Roentgen discovered X-rays in 1895 and Marie and Pierre Curie discovered the properties of radiation from radioactive isotopes such as radium and polonium in 1898. The history of using radioactive substances, particularly radium, is somewhat chequered. The report of radon-impregnated toothpaste to prevent plaque is an intriguing example of how radioactive substances were promoted in ignorance of the implications (Grigg, 1965, cited in Hilderley, 1997b). As with many things that are hailed as cure-alls of benign and malignant disease, radiation fell into disrepute with the general public in the early decades of the twentieth century.

Difficulty in replicating curative treatments was a serious problem for the developing science of radiation oncology. The principal reason for this was the lack of an accurate method to measure the dose given to the patient. From the 1900s to the 1920s, skin erythema was the most commonly used indicator of dose and treatment was given until the patient's skin could no longer tolerate the radiation. This dosage was based on the HED, the haut (skin) erythema dose, and referred to the dose required to produce a brisk skin reaction.

Despite the unscientific application of radiation and the problems of measuring dose, the science of radiation oncology continued to develop. A significant boost occurred with the development of the atomic bomb in the 1940s and the production of high-powered treatment machines such as the betatron and the linear accelerator. The cobalt teletherapy machine, which generated high-energy gamma radiation from radioactive cobalt-60, was very common in radiotherapy departments from the 1950s.

Developments over the 1950s to 1970s led to the introduction of megavoltage linear accelerators and computers to aid in the calculation of dose and accuracy of treatment. In 1953, the 'rad' was accepted as the unit of absorbed dose of any ionizing radiation. During and since this time further developments have occurred as a result of focus on clinical trials. Protocols testing radiotherapy techniques and combined protocols with other anticancer therapies have become integral to the work of many radiotherapy departments.

In 1985, the 'gray' replaced the rad as the unit of absorbed dose (1 gray = 100 rad). Further developments have been seen

over the last 20–30 years in areas such as intraoperative radiotherapy, hyperthermia and the use of radiolabelled antibodies.
Now, stereotactic radioneurosurgery using a gamma knife
provides treatment for some cranial lesions not previously accessible by standard techniques. Conformal radiotherapy and the
introduction of three-dimensional planning computers have
further enhanced the ability to increase the intensity of treatment, by reducing the volume of normal tissue within the treatment fields.

In the last two decades, a gradual shift in the organization of
radiotherapy has seen the move towards an adoption of the
team approach to care. Radiation oncology nursing has developed over this time to become integral to the care of the patient
receiving radiotherapy, and in some settings an advanced nursing role has developed.

Terminology in radiotherapy

Brachytherapy

Brachytherapy, also known as internal radiotherapy or implant
radiotherapy, is the temporary or permanent placement of a
radioactive source on or within a tumour. Brachytherapy is the
earliest therapeutic use of radiation when radium was applied to
skin lesions. The development of the linear accelerator saw
brachytherapy diminish in use over the 1960s and 1970s, but
since the 1980s interest has renewed and brachytherapy is more
commonly used. Brachytherapy can be used as the primary
treatment modality or in combination with other radiotherapy
techniques or anticancer treatments.

Brachytherapy is very commonly used for the treatment of
gynaecological cancers where a sealed source of caesium-137 is
inserted temporarily into the cervix. Another example is the use
of iodine-192, which is permanently implanted around the
prostate. The use of brachytherapy in relation to gastroenterological cancer would be for head and neck cancers, oesophageal
and rectal cancers.

Conformal radiotherapy

Conformal radiotherapy integrates computed tomography with
the radiotherapy planning computer to determine a beam
configuration that conforms precisely to the target organ or site.

Using these techniques, high-dose volumes are limited to the three-dimensional shape of the target site, thus reducing the damage to surrounding normal tissues, which results in the ability to deliver a higher dose to the target than in standard treatment.

Dosimetry

Dosimetry is the field of physics used in radiotherapy to determine the amount, rate and distribution of ionizing radiation for medicinal doses, based on body size, sex, age and other factors.

Radiopharmaceuticals

Radiopharmaceuticals are preparations of radioisotopes that can be injected into the patient. The most commonly used radiopharmaceutical is strontium-89, which is used for the palliation of metastatic bone pain. Skeletal bone metastases are a significant problem in breast, lung and prostate cancers. Strontium-89 acts like calcium in the body, clearing quickly from blood and healthy bone. It localizes selectively at sites of active osteoblastic metastasis and emits ' radiation particles selectively, sparing healthy bone (Crawford et al., 1994). Consistent pain relief occurs in the second or third week after injection and can last between 3 and 6 months, significantly reducing the need for opiate analgesia and improving the quality of life in these patients.

Simulation

Each patient who receives radiotherapy is obviously different in size and shape, and the location, size and shape of each tumour also differ. Treatment for each patient is, therefore, planned individually before it starts. Simulation is part of the planning process and involves a regular X-ray machine that is set up to simulate or mimic the exact specifications of the planned treatment. Normal radiographs are taken and the treatment plan can be checked for accuracy by radiation oncologists, physicists, radiation therapists and dosimetrists.

Teletherapy

Teletherapy, or external beam radiotherapy, is the most common treatment mode of delivering ionizing radiation. A radioactive source or electromagnetic energy from a machine external to the patient delivers the radiation. The machine is called a linear accelerator. The linear accelerator can move and be positioned at any angle around the patient. The treatment bed can be adjusted up and down, forward and back, and also around in a circle. The combination of all these movements means that the beam of radiation can be directed at any part of the body as required. Linear accelerators emit varying types of energy that have differing characteristics and radiobiological effect. A considerable amount has been written on the technical aspects of teletherapy, e.g. Hilderley (1997c) and Perez and Brady (1997).

Indications for radiotherapy

Curative radiotherapy

As stated, radiotherapy can be used alone or in combination with other anticancer therapies when the goal of treatment is for cure (radical radiotherapy), or to control cancer or palliate symptoms (palliative radiotherapy). Radiotherapy is a localized treatment so, for a cure to be achieved, some conditions need to be met which are:

- Radiosensitive tumours that are relatively localized
- A high growth factor (high percentage of cells in active division)
- Location of tumour (proximity to vital structures)
- Extent of metastases (distant metastases limit effectiveness).

Some tumour types are more responsive to ionizing radiation than others; this is called radiosensitivity. A familiar analogy would be that some micro-organisms are more sensitive to a particular antibiotic. To achieve a cure, a tumour that is localized (there is no spread to surrounding tissue) and sensitive to the effects of ionizing radiation will be more curable.

Radiotherapy affects cells as only they go through active mitosis, so a higher growth factor in the tumour reflects more cells in active mitosis. This is explained further later in the chapter. Normal (non-malignant) tissues have different tolerances to ionizing radiation, depending on their cell type. The more specialized a cell type is, the lower the tolerance to radiation, because the healing ability of those cell types is limited, e.g.

spinal cord has a very low tolerance to radiation, as does lung, liver and kidney tissue.

If there is evidence of a distant metastasis, the effectiveness of radiotherapy achieving a cure is limited because of the localized nature of the treatment. Metastatic disease indicates that the cancer is systemic rather than localized, and requires systemic treatment in the form of chemotherapy.

Palliative radiotherapy

About 70% of the work of most radiotherapy departments could be considered palliative. Indications for palliative radiotherapy are:

- pain
- compression of vital structures (e.g. brain, spinal cord, superior vena cava)
- malignant effusion
- bony metastases
- brain secondaries
- malignant ulcers (fungating tumours).

What happens to the patient?

Although there are standardized protocols for the delivery of radiotherapy, each patient is different in shape, size and location of the tumour, so an individual approach to treatment is taken. After consultation the decision to go ahead is made. A second appointment is scheduled to plan treatment. A planning appointment takes longer than treatment and may last 30–60 minutes. The patient is positioned on the treatment couch exactly as he or she will lie during treatment. A simulator takes normal radiographs of the treatment location and from that an accurate treatment plan is marked and calculated. To assist with daily set-up of the linear accelerator, the patient's skin is marked with chinagraph pencil, gentian violet or marker pen, or pinprick tattoos are made. The planning process is not painful in itself; however, if patients will be in pain from lying in bed in one position for extended periods, it is important to ensure adequate prior analgesia.

Treatment with external beam radiotherapy usually occurs daily, Monday to Friday, with an appointment time at about the same time each day. Treatment takes only a few minutes each visit. Usually once a week, the patient will be reviewed by the clinical oncologist; however, it is important to remind patients that there is always a nurse available to discuss problems at any time.

Introduction to radiobiology

Radiotherapy is a local treatment for cancer, so the actions and reactions to radiotherapy are confined entirely to the treatment fields (area being treated). The notable exception to this is fatigue. Fatigue is the only systemic effect of radiotherapy and its management is discussed in Chapter 10.

The aim of radiotherapy is described by Perez and Brady (1997, p 1.) as follows:

> To deliver a precisely measured dose of ionising radiation to a defined tumour volume with as minimal damage as possible to surrounding healthy tissue, resulting in the eradication of the tumour, a high quality of life, and prolongation of survival at reasonable cost.

The importance of this objective lies in the fact that radiation affects all living cells, both malignant and normal. A balance between the destruction of malignant cells and the preservation of normal cells must be maintained in order to achieve the best possible results for the patient with cancer.

The cell can be damaged by ionizing radiation directly, through immediate damage to DNA synthesis, or indirectly, through the production of free radicals in the cell. The mechanism of damage occurs at the cellular level and is intimately connected with the process of replication. The process of replication is similar for both normal and malignant cells and comprises a progression through four distinct phases known as the cell cycle. Figure 8.1 illustrates the phases and briefly outlines the functions of each phase.

The cell is most vulnerable to direct damage from ionizing radiation during the phases of the cell cycle when DNA synthesis or mitosis can be disrupted. Specifically, radiation damage affects the following three phases: G1, when substances necessary for DNA synthesis are altered; G2, when protein synthesis is inhibited and changes occur in the chromosomes; and during mitosis, when the altered chromosomes lose their ability to reproduce (Figure 8.1).

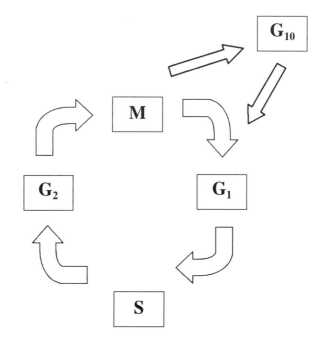

Figure 8.1 Phases of cell cycle.

However, the primary cause of damage is induced by the ionization events derived from the indirect action of radiation, because, at the moment of irradiation, most cells are more likely to be in cell cycle phases other than active mitosis. The cellular response to radiation involves the creation of free radicals in the cell by the interaction of cell water and electrons ejected from atomic structures after passage of radiation through the cell. Free radicals alter the atomic and molecular structures, damaging the DNA in the cell nucleus. It is estimated that about 70% of the biological damage produced by X-rays is the result of the indirect action mediated by free radicals (Hall, 1985). The presence of oxygen acts as a sensitizer in the cell, causing further damage to DNA through the formation of oxidizing substances, such as hydrogen peroxide, which occurs when oxygen reacts with free radicals (Holmes, 1988; Hilderley, 1993). Ultimately the effects of radiation, whether direct or indirect, damage the cell's DNA, leading to the inhibition or failure of mitosis. Depending on the radiation dose, cell death may occur immediately or within hours, but is usually preceded by one or more cell cycles after radiation (Hilderley, 1993).

Fractionation

Given that all cells, whether malignant or normal, are damaged by ionizing radiation, it is important to understand the ways in which the delivery of radiotherapy minimizes the damage to normal cells. The principal method for this is dose fractionation. Fractionation is the division of the total dose of radiation into smaller doses (fractions) and the advantage gained is based on the four Rs of radiotherapy: repopulation, redistribution, repair and reoxygenation. These four basic factors are considered to be the mechanisms by which fractionation improves tumour eradication and minimizes normal tissue damage (Withers, 1992; Hilderley, 1993).

Repopulation

Germinal cells of the skin and mucous membranes show an early regenerative response through increased rates of cell proliferation. Repopulation may begin before the course of radiotherapy has ended and, as with the physiological response to any trauma, the repopulation rate accelerates, creating what is termed an 'avalanche effect' (Withers, 1992).

Fractionation is assumed to have a protective effect on the normal tissues. The assumption is limited, however, by the fact that repopulation of cells may occur over a prolonged period (Fowler, 1979). If the overall treatment time is over-extended or interrupted unexpectedly, the extra time between fractions or any time off treatment allows regeneration of tumour cells as well as normal cells. To achieve optimal tumour eradication, additional fractions would be required, resulting in a higher total dose. A higher total dose has implications for the overall normal tissue damage in both the acute and the chronic phases. The optimal effect is achieved by planning for the overall treatment time to be as short as possible.

Redistribution

As already stated, the effect on tumour eradication can be enhanced if the treatment is given over a shorter time. This effect is enhanced if smaller, more frequent fractions are also given, e.g. two or more times per day (hyperfractionation) and further still if treatment is given 6 or 7 days per week instead of the standard 5 (accelerated hyperfractionation). Cells vary in their radiosensitivity as they move through the phases of the cell cycle, with the greatest radiosensitivity for direct damage occurring in the late S-phase and the G2–M phase. After each fraction of radiation, surviving cells, which are in relatively radiation-resistant phases of the cell cycle, progress to more sensitive phases. The net gain in this process, in terms of tumour eradication, is that cells 'self-sensitize', resulting in more cells reaching the mitotic phase as the next dose is given (Withers, 1992; Hilderley, 1993). Protocols exploiting this phenomenon are the subject of current clinical trials and redistribution is the mechanism thought to be responsible.

Redistribution is a phenomenon of acute responding tissues (such as tumour, and normal skin, mucosa and bone marrow) and not of late responding tissues (such as spinal cord, brain or kidney). Therefore, hyperfractionation exacerbates acute effects, but reduces, theoretically, the late effects. Combining radiation with chemotherapeutic agents, such as methotrexate and hydroxyurea, is proving to be another method of exploiting redistribution (Hilderley, 1993).

Repair

The ability of the cell to repair after each fraction of radiation is the key to the survival of acute responding normal tissues. Withers (1992) cites research from as long ago as 1959 which showed that cells could be repaired after radiation, given a few hours of normal metabolic activity.

Repair is initiated by the body immediately and continues in acute responding tissues for 3–4 hours after each fraction of radiation. Tumour cells also can repair between fractions, but the assumption underlying all radiation treatment is that less repair of radiation damage occurs in tumour cells than in normal tissues. In addition, reoxygenation further radiosensitizes the tumour, resulting in improved tumour kill when the next fraction is given.

Reoxygenation

As discussed previously, oxygen is necessary for the production of some free radicals important in the mechanism for indirect damage to DNA. Hypoxia therefore causes the cellular response to radiation to be reduced (Holmes, 1988). The importance of oxygen concentration at the time of radiotherapy has been known for over 60 years (Hall, 1985). In the laboratory it has been shown that the dose required to eradicate all tumour cells may be doubled where just 2–3% of the cells are hypoxic (Gray et al., 1953; Dische, 1991). As a result, studies have been undertaken to identify methods to increase the radiosensitivity of hypoxic tumour cells. Reoxygenation occurs after each fraction of radiation as part of the body's normal tissue repair process. Fractionation therefore optimizes the reoxygenation process by increasing the oxygen concentration in the tumour.

The effect of radiotherapy on normal tissue

The skin and mucosa perform an important function in the protective mechanisms of the body, providing a specialized covering based on an epithelial outer layer and a deeper connective tissue layer. The health of the skin and mucosa and the body's ability to repair damage significantly affect the quality of life of patients undergoing anticancer treatment. Skin and mucosal reactions are particularly important to understand in relation to the patient with gastrointestinal cancer; the following discussion focuses primarily on these side effects.

The best way to think about the effects of radiation on skin and mucosa is in terms of radiation being a physical trauma causing cell damage or death just as any other trauma such as a burn or cut. The body's normal response to trauma is through the inflammatory response. Acute radiation skin and mucosal reactions are no different. The irradiated skin becomes inflamed and heat, pain, oedema and erythema are observed. Evidence that the tissue has been damaged cannot be seen immediately because the damage has occurred at the basal cell layer where replication takes place. Therefore the first sign of a skin reaction is at 10–14 days – the time it takes for the damaged cells to migrate to the outer layer of the epidermis. The time taken for mucosal reactions is a little shorter.

All cells/tissue in the direct field of the radiation will be affected by ionization. Cells that have a rapid turnover will exhibit acute reactions during the treatment period. These tissue types include skin, mucosa, hair follicles, sweat and salivary glands, and bone marrow. Cells that have a slower turnover, such as lung or connective tissue, exhibit damage later, often months or even years after treatment, and these represent the late effects of treatment. All radiation damage ultimately becomes chronic in nature and care of the skin and gut mucosa is discussed later.

Recovery and healing can and do occur between the fractions of radiotherapy, which is why several hours (usually 6–8 hours) must pass before additional fractions can be given. Healing and repair also continue to occur after treatment.

Management of acute radiation: skin and mucosal reactions

Many people, patients and health professionals alike, in recognition of the fact that radiotherapy is a complex and unfamiliar treatment, think that the management of skin reactions and other side effects is equally complex and, as a result, anxiety provoking. However, by remembering two important facts, the care of the patient's skin can be deduced logically. The first is that ionizing radiation damages cells during mitosis only and the second is that the body's response mechanism to radiation is the same as for any physical trauma – the inflammatory response.

Using the skin as the model for understanding all radiation reactions, the germinal layer (stratum germinativum) is the site of damage. The skin reaction manifests as erythema 10–14 days after the first fraction of radiation, because this is the transit time for new skin cells to migrate to the surface, transforming through the skin layers to form the dead outer layer, the stratum corneum. Germinal cells multiply more frequently to replace damaged cells, so the cells that migrate to become the stratum corneum are more vulnerable to normal wear and tear on the skin surface. As a result, dry desquamation (peeling) occurs. If the damage is more extensive, the epidermis sloughs producing moist desquamation.

The cardinal signs of inflammation become evident as the skin reaction develops: erythema, oedema, tenderness and heat. The appearance of the skin is often described as similar to sunburn with peeling (dry desquamation) and itching. The reaction may become more severe with varying degrees of epidermal loss (moist desquamation) and, on extremely rare occasions, necrosis. Discomfort ranges from mildly irritating to severe pain. Skin reactions can be graded; two well-used measures are the Radiation Therapy Oncology Group (RTOG) Acute Reaction Scoring System (Cox et al., 1995) and the Oncology Nursing Society scoring (Blackmar and Bull-Hurst, 1994) (Tables 8.1 and 8.2).

Table 8.1 Radiation Therapy Oncology Group (RTOG) score system for acute radiation skin reactions

RTOG* scores			
1	2	3	4
Follicular, faint or dull erythema, epilation, dry desquamation, decreased sweating	Tender or bright erythema, patchy moist desquamation, moderate oedema	Confluent, moist desquamation other than skin folds, pitting oedema	Ulceration, haemorrhage, necrosis

*RTOG score of 0 = no change over baseline.

Table 8.2 Oncology Nursing Society radiation skin reaction scoring system

Score	Description
0	No changes noted
1	Faint or dull erythema, follicular reaction
2	Bright erythema
3	Dry desquamation with or without erythema
4	Small-to-moderate wet desquamation
5	Confluent moist desquamation
6	Ulceration, haemorrhage or necrosis

Skin that has been irradiated will be changed permanently, but it will still function adequately under normal circumstances. As might be expected when the effects of inflammation occur over several weeks, scarring and fibrosis occur as a late effect of treatment with radiation. An old radiation site takes on a typical appearance with loss of pigmentation (resulting from destruction of melanocytes), indentation (caused by fibrosis of collagen and supporting structures in the dermis) and telangiectasis, which appears as spidery red lines across the skin surface (as a result of fibrosis of the blood vessels). These permanent fibrotic changes result in the area being prone to poor healing. It is therefore wise to remember that irradiated skin, no matter how long ago it was irradiated, should always be treated with care, in particular avoiding any trauma.

There is little empirical evidence on which to base guidelines for skin care during treatment, the choice of topical agents or dressings for the management of radiation skin reactions. As a result, the skin care may vary considerably between institutions and practitioners – an issue that has been raised by a number of authors (Thomas, 1992; Barkham, 1993; Lavery, 1995; Campbell and Lanec, 1996; Blackmar, 1997). The purpose of managing the inevitable damage caused by radiation to the skin is therefore to minimize the effects, wherever possible, and at all times help to keep the patient comfortable.

Guidelines for skin care during radiotherapy

The aim of skin care guidelines is to maintain the stratum corneum intact for as long as possible. This is achieved by reducing undue irritation or trauma to the irradiated skin. Restriction of harsh soaps, deodorants or perfumes in the treated area is usually suggested. Soft, loose, cotton clothing is also recommended, as is protecting the area from the elements and extremes of temperature. In addition topical agents that contain metals are contraindicated because they accumulate the dose of radiation at the skin level. Examples of products containing metals are zinc and castor oil cream or deodorants, which often contain aluminium. It should be noted that the restrictions apply only to the immediate area of the radiation field.

There is still some controversy over whether patients should wash the treatment area with soap and water, water alone or not at all. Two reasons for not washing the skin in the treatment area have been generally reported. First, there was the belief that the skin should not be touched in case the patient inadvertently rubbed the skin too harshly. Second, 'the marks' drawn on the skin with a chinagraph pencil to assist radiation therapists' set-up for the treatment each day would be removed. However, modern techniques for setting up treatment each day now mean that marks can be removed before the patient leaves the department. Also, pinprick tattoos are more frequently used to ensure the accuracy of landmarks, removing the necessity for some drawn marks.

With regard to the washing of the radiation site, all research that has tested washing guidelines has reported no worsening of the skin reaction when soap and water are used. Campbell and Illingworth (1992) conducted a randomized trial of 99 patients receiving radiotherapy to the breast or chest wall. The findings showed no significant differences among three groups of patients who washed with water alone or with soap and water, or did not wash the area. In addition, subjective evidence showed that skin reactions were less severe in the two washing groups than the group that was not permitted to wash at all.

More recently, a study of women treated for breast cancer found no difference in the severity of skin reactions between women who followed the convention of washing with water only during treatment and those who maintained their usual hygiene regimen (Meegan and Haycocks, 1997).

The evidence would therefore suggest that gentle washing with water and a mild soap will not damage the skin and will probably help the patient to feel more comfortable. Clinical experience certainly supports the notion that patients feel better and are more comfortable when treatment areas are washed gently with a moisturized soap. It is important to emphasize to patients that they just pat the skin dry with a soft towel to prevent excessive rubbing, even when the area is itchy.

Several papers have been published as educational resources for nurses to assist them in making clinical decisions about topical treatment of radiation skin reactions. These papers suggest the use of light creams, ointments and steroids to moisturize the skin when erythema or dry desquamation occurs (McDonald, 1992; Sitton, 1992; Barkham, 1993; Campbell and Lanec, 1996; Blackmar, 1997; Porock and Kristjanson, 1999). However, there is a paucity of empirical evidence to support the use of creams to prevent the development of radiation skin reactions or promote healing. In addition, the topical agents tested are not necessarily the ones commonly used in clinical practice.

A randomized controlled trial of sucralfate cream versus a placebo made with the same base cream was conducted during electron beam therapy to the lumpectomy scars of 50 women treated for breast cancer (Maiche et al., 1994). Unfortunately, no details were reported on the reliability of skin reaction measures. Results showed that early erythema appeared later and recovery was significantly faster in the area treated with sucralfate cream. This study provides some fairly convincing evidence of the benefits of sucralfate cream and discusses the possible mechanisms of action.

Another less familiar treatment, camomile cream, was tested against almond ointment, which was described as the standard treatment in the study department in Sweden. In this observer-masked randomized trial, 48 women being treated for breast cancer applied both agents to the radiation site, choosing which half of the area would receive the camomile cream. Almond ointment was applied to the remaining area. At the end of the treatment period, there was no statistically significant difference in the severity of the skin reaction between the two creams. However, the skin reaction where the camomile was used appeared later and the patients preferred the camomile cream to the almond ointment. Interestingly only five cases of moist desquamation were reported in the camomile-treated areas, whereas 13 were reported in the almond ointment-treated areas. There is no indication whether these were the same patients, i.e. whether the patient was particularly prone to a more severe skin reaction.

Aloe vera is frequently advocated in the lay press as a natural ointment for promoting wound healing. Consequently, it is not uncommon for patients to ask if they can use aloe vera on their skin during radiotherapy. The literature is divided on the efficacy of this product. The best evidence located was the report of two randomized, controlled trials (Williams et al., 1996). The first was a double-masked trial with aloe vera versus a placebo gel in 194 women receiving breast or chest wall radiation. The second randomized 108 such patients to aloe vera gel versus no treatment. Radiation reactions were virtually identical in both treatment groups in both trials. The conclusion offered by Williams and colleagues was that aloe vera gel does not protect against radiation-induced injury. Nevertheless, anecdotal reports from patients continue to support the notion that aloe vera aids healing, so research continues. A small, unpublished, pilot study in Queensland investigated the effect of aloe vera versus aqueous cream (S Toye, personal communication, July 1998). A trend emerged showing that the application of aloe vera three times a day was more effective than aqueous cream in reducing itching, erythema pain and skin breakdown. A phase III trial is continuing. Toye's pilot study did show that aqueous cream was more effective in managing dry desquamation than aloe vera. The usefulness of aqueous cream for dry desquamation is supported in Porock and Kristjanson's (1999) findings.

A trial of Bepanthen versus no cream was conducted on 63 breast and 16 laryngeal cancer patients (Løkkevik et al., 1996). Bepanthen was applied to approximately half of the treatment area, with the patient randomly selecting the area treated. The evaluating physician was unaware of which half of the skin reaction the patient was treating with Bepanthen. Significant differences were found in the mild reactions, with Bepanthen reducing the skin reaction. However, for patients who developed a reaction of severe erythema developing into patchy moist desquamation, there was no significant difference between using no cream and using Bepanthen. Worse reactions were reported in about 10% of the sample in terms of erythema, desquamation, itch and pain. Porock and Kristjanson (1999) did not report the exacerbation of skin reactions with Bepanthen; however, the finding that there was no evidence to suggest that Bepanthen promoted healing was corroborated.

Where moist desquamation occurs there is some contention as to the best method to manage this problem. In the past, the recommended course of action was to cleanse the area with half-strength hydrogen peroxide and physiological (0.9%) saline and then paint with 1% gentian violet solution (Holmes, 1988). Hydrogen peroxide has long been disputed as an appropriate solution for cleaning wounds; in line with this, the best solution for cleansing the area of moist desquamation is 0.9% saline or gently washing with warm tap water and mild soap. It is important to warm the cleansing solution because areas of moist desquamation are generally very sensitive to cold and warming the solution helps reduce the discomfort.

The benefits of gentian violet were thought to be from its antibacterial/antifungal action. However, its use is no longer recommended for open wounds or mucous membranes because animal studies have shown gentian violet to be carcinogenic (Littlefield et al., 1985; DHSS, 1987; BMA/RPSGB, 1994). Given the current knowledge of wound healing and management of wounds that are infected, the best course of action is to treat the patient systemically rather than with topical agents (Dealey, 1994; Carville, 1995).

During treatment, dressings must be removed because they interfere with the set-up of the radiotherapy. It is very important that the dressing materials used to cover and protect an area of moist desquamation will not stick to the wound because the risk of removing newly granulating tissue is high, thereby increasing the risk of radionecrotic ulcer formation. Petroleum jelly (Vaseline)-impregnated gauze is useful, but can still dry out and stick to the newly granulating wound bed. The addition of sterilized plain emollient to the dressing before its placement on the wound will help prevent trauma to the wound on removal of the dressing before treatment. This can be further covered with cotton-wool gauze pads to provide protection against friction. Alternatives to adhesive dressing tapes must be found to prevent further trauma in the irradiated area, e.g. tubular bandages.

An exception to the rule of removing all dressing materials during treatment can be found in a case study report of retention tape (e.g. Fixomull and Hypafix) being used as a dressing (Downes et al., 1997). The case studies showed that the use of retention tape, in a similar way to its use in donor site dressings, promoted healing and comfort for patients with moist desquamation. The mechanism for healing was suggested to be that the retention tape created an artificial stratum corneum, protecting the new, vulnerable skin from additional trauma and infection.

Once treatment is complete, application of the principles of moist wound healing, using a variety of dressing materials is appropriate. Some work has begun on testing these dressings with moist desquamation; overall the findings are inconclusive.

A report on the use of a hydrocolloid dressing in 18 patients with moist desquamation indicated the benefits in terms of healing time, comfort and aesthetics (Margolin et al., 1990). The sites used for the dressing were not reported and neither was the dose of radiation. Although these results are encouraging, lack of a comparison group and the small sample size limit the clinical recommendations that can be made based on this study.

Shell et al. (1986) reported on a study of 16 patients with dry and moist desquamation where a moisture vapour-permeable (MVP) dressing was compared with conventional dressings of hydrous lanolin gauze. Radiation skin reactions were located on the head and neck, chest or back. Results from this small sample showed a trend towards faster healing time for the MVP dressing and a reduction in discomfort. Again the evidence was inconclusive.

The theory of moist wound healing (Westaby, 1985) provides the rationale for tests of various dressing materials reported in empirical research and case studies. This theoretical base strengthens the evidence that dressing materials have an important role in promoting healing of moist desquamation. However, evidence to date on topical agents is much less convincing.

Acute radiation mucosal reactions

Mucosal reactions follow a very similar course to skin reactions, although the temptation to apply creams and dressings is somewhat removed. Table 8.3 provides an assessment for all gut mucosal reactions. As with skin reactions, quality assessment is the key to improving symptom management in mucosal reactions. To reduce the friction and soreness associated particularly

Table 8.3 Radiation Therapy Oncology Group (RTOG) toxicity for acute mucosal reactions

Site of reaction	RTOG scores*			
	1	2	3	4
Mucous membranes	Injection, may experience mild pain not requiring analgesia	Patchy mucositis may produce an inflammatory serosanguineous discharge; may experience moderate pain requiring analgesia	Confluent fibrinous mucositis may include severe pain requiring opiate	Ulceration, haemorrhage, necrosis
Salivary gland	Mild mouth dryness, slightly thickened saliva; may have altered taste such as metallic; these changes not reflected in baseline feeding such as increased liquids with meals			Acute salivary gland necrosis
Pharynx	Mild dysphagia may require topical anaesthetic or non-opiate analgesia; may require soft diet	Moderate dysphagia may require opiate analgesia; may require purée or liquid diet	Severe dysphagia with dehydration or weight loss requiring nasogastric tube feeding, intravenous fluids or hyperalimentation	Complete obstruction, ulceration, perforation, fistula
Larynx	Mild or intermittent hoarseness, cough not requiring anti-tussive; erythema of mucosa	Persistent hoarseness but able to vocalize; referred ear pain, sore throat, patchy fibrinous exudate or mild erythroid oedema not requiring opiate, cough requiring anti-tussive	Whispered speech throat pain or referred ear pain requiring opiate. Confluent fibrinous exudate, marked erythroid oedema	Marked dyspnoea, stridor or haemoptysis with tracheostomy or intubation

*RTOG score of 0 = no change over baseline.

with oral mucosal reactions, foods that are soft, not spicy and not rough are recommended. Several preparations for increasing comfort, and thus promoting eating, include local anaesthetic preparations to be used before meal times.

Oral, pharyngeal and laryngeal reactions

In the oral mucosa the salivary glands are damaged, causing a reduction in or complete inhibition of the production of saliva. Xerostomia (dry mouth resulting from absence of saliva) in the oral mucosa is a particularly uncomfortable and distressing side effect of treatment, which occurs if the parotid glands are in the treatment field.

Upper GI mucosal reactions

Oesophagitis is the principal complaint of patients who have the upper GI treated. Mucosal sloughing makes the ingestion of food very difficult and is not easy to overcome. Other than the restriction of spicy or hot food, the main symptomatic treatment is to use antacid preparations that contain a local anaesthetic. This, if swallowed 5–10 minutes before eating, can reduce the discomfort of food passing down the oesophagus. Another tip is to instruct the patient to take small mouthfuls and swallow small amounts at a time to prevent unnecessary distension of the oesophagus. Drinking fluid with the meal or eating soft or moist foods may also help.

Lower GI mucosal reactions

The principal side effect from lower GI radiotherapy is diarrhoea. The fluidity, consistency, urgency and frequency depend on the area of the bowel being treated. For patients undergoing rectal radiotherapy an additional problem can be proctitis; this often causes a great deal of distress and discomfort. Traditionally, a low-residue (low-fibre) diet has been prescribed for radiation to the bowel. However, more recent research by Faithfull et al. (2001) suggests that this is not a logical solution to the problem.

Management of chronic radiation: skin and mucosal reactions

Principles of chronic management

The long-term effects of radiotherapy on normal tissue are fibrosis, which occurs as a result of the scarring left from severe inflammation. All the tissues in the field of radiotherapy will become fibrotic, including blood vessels, connective tissue, melanocytes, hair follicles and sweat, sebaceous and salivary glands. This gives the skin and mucosa a typical appearance. The skin, for example, becomes indented (as a result of loss of connective tissue), loses pigmentation (caused by fibrosis of melanocytes) and telangiectases appear (resulting from fibrosis of blood vessels).

Although the skin will function adequately despite these chronic effects of radiotherapy, it is particularly vulnerable to damage. Healing is slow as a result of poor replication and fibrotic blood vessels being unable to transport oxygen and nutrients readily to the damaged area. Furthermore, if radiation affected lymph tissue, the removal of debris is also impaired, which also slows healing. In the worst cases, damage to a chronic radiation skin or mucosal reaction can cause a radionecrotic ulcer to form which may not heal.

To care for skin that has been irradiated, it should be moisturized to prevent excessive dryness and peeling, it should be protected from the sun and extreme elements, and care should be taken to prevent skin breakdown. Chronic mucosal reactions can be seen with endoscopy and care should be taken to avoid damaging the mucosa during the procedure as healing will be slow and potentially painful.

Conclusion

Radiotherapy is a common treatment for cancer but is often not well understood by health professionals or patients. Simple guidelines based on the understanding of basic principles of radiation can help provide comfort and support to patients undergoing radiotherapy. Care of the skin and mucous membranes is an important aspect of the nursing role not only during the treatment period but also in long-term follow-up.

References

American Cancer Society (1996) Cancer Facts and Figures. Atlanta, GA: American Cancer Society.

Barkham AM (1993) Radiotherapy skin reactions. Professional Nurs. August: 732-736.

Blackmar A (1997) Radiation-induced skin alterations, Focus on Wound Care 6: 172-175.

Blackmar A, Bull-Hurst T (1994) Radiation Therapy Documentation. Pittsburgh, PA: Oncology Nursing Society.

British Medical Association and Royal Pharmacological Society of Great Britain (1994) British National Formulary, Number 27. London: BMA/RPSGP.

Calman K, Hine D (1995) A Policy Framework for Commissioning Cancer Services: A Report by the Expert Advisory Group on Cancer to the Chief Medical Officers of England and Wales. London: Department of Health.

Campbell IR, Illingworth MH (1992) Can patients wash during radiotherapy to the breast or chest wall? A randomized controlled trial. Clinical Oncology 4: 78–82.

Campbell J, Lanec C (1996) Developing a skin-care protocol in radiotherapy. Professional Nurse 12: 105–108.

Carville K (1995) Wound Care Manual, revised edn. Western Australia: Silver Chain Foundation.

Cox JD, Stetz J, Pajak TF (1995) Toxicity criteria of the Radiation Therapy Oncology Group (RTOG) and the European Organization for Research and Treatment of Cancer (EORTC) International Journal of Radiation Oncology, Biology, Physics 31: 1341–1346.

Crawford E, Kozlowski, J, Debruyne F et al. (1994) The use of strontium-89 for palliation of pain from bone metastases associated with hormone-refractory prostate cancer. Urology 44: 481–485.

Dealey C (1994) The Care of Wounds: A guide for nurse.s Oxford: Blackwell Scientific Publications.

Department of Health and Social Services (DHSS) (1987) Restriction on the use of crystal violet. Pharmacology Journal 289: 665.

Dische S (1991) A review of hypoxic cell radiosensitization. International Journal of Radiation Oncology, Biology, Physics 20: 147–152.

Downes M, Porock D, Upright C (1997) Retention dressings: An alternative for patient comfort in radiation skin reactions. Primary Intention 5: 16–22.

Faithfull S, Corner J, Meyer L, Huddart R, Dearnaley D (2001) Evaluation of nurse-led follow up for patients undergoing pelvic radiotherapy. British Journal of Cancer 85: 1853–1864.

Fowler JF (1979) New horizons in radiation oncology. British Journal of Radiology 52: 523–535.

Gray LH, Conger AD, Ebert M, Hornsey S, Scott OCA (1953) The concentration of oxygen dissolved in tissues at the time of irradiation as a factor in radiotherapy. British Journal of Radiology 26: 638–648.

Hall EJ (1985) Radiation biology. Cancer 55: 2051–2057.

Hilderley LJ (1993) Radiotherapy. In Groenwald SL, Frogge MH, Goodman M, Yarbro CH (eds), Cancer Nursing. Principles and practice, 3rd edn. Boston: Jones & Bartlett.

Hilderley LJ (1997a) Principles of teletherapy. In: Dow KH, Hilderley LJ (eds), Nursing Care in Radiation Oncology, 2nd edn. Philadelphia: WB Saunders, pp. 3–5.

Hilderley LJ (1997b) Radiation oncology: historical background. In: Dow KH et al. (eds), Nursing Care in Radiation Oncology, 2nd edn. Philadelphia: WB Saunders, pp. 3–5.

Hilderley LJ (1997c) Radiotherapy. In: Groenwald SL, Frogge MH, Goodman M, Yarbro CH (eds), Cancer Nursing. Principles and practice, 4th edn. Boston: Jones & Bartlett, pp. 47–283.

Holmes S (1988) Radiotherapy. London: Austin Cornish.

Lavery BA (1995) Skin care during radiotherapy: a survey of UK practice. Clinical Oncology 7: 184–187.

Littlefield NA, Blackwell B, Hewitt CC, Gaylor DW (1985) Chronic toxicity and carcinogenicity studies of gentian violet in mice. Fundamental and Applied Toxicology 5: 902–912.

Løkkevik E, Skovlund E, Reitan J B, Hannisdal E, Tanum G (1996) Skin treatment with Bepanthen cream versus no cream during radiotherapy. Acta Oncologica 35: 1021–1026.

McDonald A (1992) Altered protective mechanisms. In: Dow KH, Hilderley LJ (eds), Nursing Care in Radiation Oncology. Philadelphia, PA: WB Saunders Co., pp. 79–96.

Maiche A, Isokangas O, Gröhn P (1994) Skin protection by sucralfate cream during electron beam therapy. Acta Oncologica 33: 201–203.

Margolin SG, Breneman JC, Denman DL, LaChapelle P, Weckbach, L, Aron BS (1990) Management of radiation-induced moist skin desquamation using hydrocolloid dressing. Cancer Nursing 13: 71–80.

Meegan MA, Haycocks TR (1997) An investigation into the management of acute skin infections from tangential breast irradiation. Canadian Journal of Medical Technology 28: 169–173.

Perez CA, Brady LW (1997) Principles and Practice of Radiation Oncology, 3rd edn. Philadelphia, PA: JB Lippincott Co

Porock D, Kristjanson L (1999) Skin reactions during radiotherapy for breast cancer: the use and impact of topical agents and dressings. European Journal of Cancer Care 8: 143–153.

Shell JA, Stanutz F, Grimm J (1986) Comparison of moisture vapor permeable (MVP) dressings for management of radiation skin reactions. Oncology Nursing Forum 13: 11–16.

Sitton E (1992) Early and late radiation-induced skin alterations. Part 1: Mechanisms of skin changes. Oncology Nursing Forum 19: 801–807.

Thomas S (1992) Current Practices in the Management of Fungating Lesions and Radiation Damaged Skin. Bridgend: Surgical Materials Testing Laboratory.

Westaby G (1985) Wound Care. London: William Heinemann Medical Books Ltd.

Withers HJ (1992) Biologic basis of radiation therapy. In: Perez CA, Brady LW (eds), Principles and Practice of Radiation Oncology, 2nd edn. Philadelphia, PA: JB Lippincott Co., pp. 64–96.

Williams M, Burk M, Loprinzi M et al. (1996) Phase III double-blind evaluation of an aloe vera gel as a prophylactic agent for radiation-induced skin toxicity. International Journal of Radiation Oncology 36: 345–349.

CHAPTER 9

Care of the patient receiving chemotherapy

SALLY LEGGE

The aim of this chapter is to give the nurse a clear understanding of the chemotherapy agents used in the treatment of gastrointestinal cancers and the nursing care involved. The areas discussed include:

- An overview of the cell cycle
- Drug resistance
- Clinical determinants and the use of chemotherapy
- The role of chemotherapy in the treatment of gastrointestinal tumours
- The nursing role and the patient's experience
- Nursing care of intravenous devices and the handling of chemotherapy
- Nursing management of chemotherapy-induced side effects
- Patient selection criteria
- The role of clinical trials
- Patient information/education.

Overview of the cell cycle and action of cytotoxic agents

Cytotoxic agents interfere with cell replication, which brings about tumour death or tumour stasis (Wilkes, 1996). However, cytotoxics attack dividing cells, normal or abnormal, causing side effects. All cells replicate following specific phases (Holmes, 1990 a and b):

G1: RNA and protein synthesis occurs in preparation for DNA synthesis
S: DNA synthesis occurs, preparing for cell division

G2: RNA and specific proteins are synthesized which are neces-
     sary for mitosis
M: mitosis occurs
G0: a resting phase outside of the cell cycle; the cell is unable to
     divide until it is stimulated to return to the cell cycle

Cytotoxic agents either attack cells at cell cycle-specific phases
(phase specific) or are indiscriminate to any particular phase (cell
cycle non-specific). Cell destruction is caused by direct interference with DNA, through interference with the enzymes needed
for DNA or RNA synthesis or by destruction of the cellular
proteins needed for DNA production. The combination of different cytotoxic agents within a regimen has the advantage of a
multi-phase attack on the cell cycle, resulting in improved tumour
lysis (destruction). Below is an example of the mechanism of 5-
fluorouracil (5FU), the most commonly used agent for gastrointestinal cancer, which is known to have three predominant
intracellular mechanisms of action (Meropol et al., 1995):

1. 5FU is converted into fluorodeoxyuridine monophosphate
   (FdUMP), which binds with thymidylate synthase (TS), an
   enzyme necessary for DNA synthesis; this results in cell
   destruction.
2. 5FU is also converted into a substance, fluorouridine triphos-
   phate (FUTP), that is incorporated into RNA and interferes
   with normal RNA function.
3. DNA stability is also altered by fluorodeoxyuridine triphos-
   phate (FdUTP)

The cytotoxic mechanism of 5FU differs depending on the
method of administration, which may be via an intravenous
route or an oral preparation; the latter is still undergoing clinical
trials. One such oral fluoropyrimidine, Capecitabine (Xeloda), is
metabolised to 5FU with the help of thymidine phosphorylase
(TP). Thymidine phosphorlase, a platlet derived endothelial cell
growth factor is significantly more active in tumour tissue than
healthy tissue. This results in Capecitabine having a greater
tumour selectivity (Van Cutsem et al., 2001). Intravenous administration may be as single-dose intravenous injection, consecu-
tive-day bolus injections, short (48-hour) or protracted
infusions. 5FU is S-phase specific and has a short half-life of
approximately 20 minutes. Therefore, protracted infusions can

increase the potential of cellular damage. Allegra and Grem (1997) demonstrated that the presence of 5FU enhanced the cytotoxicity of ionizing radiation and that protracted infusion of 5FU was very effective. Concomitant chemoradiation has now been incorporated into clinical trials.

Drug resistance

Drug resistance is a major obstacle to achieving the goal of curing cancer (Beck and Dalton, 1997). The mechanisms of drug resistance are complex. One of the significant causes of multidrug resistance is the presence of P-glycoprotein in the cell, which acts actively to drive out the drug. Multidrug resistance can occur with cell exposure to a single chemotherapeutic agent, particularly those derived from natural products (Ingwersen, 1996). The lower gastrointestinal tract and the liver are also thought to be affected by high levels of enzymes known as GSTs (glutathione-s-transferase) which aid in the repair of damaged DNA. This results in an increased resistance to certain types of cytotoxic agents (Ahlgren, 1992). Drug resistance is related to many factors (Ingwersen, 1996; Beck and Dalton, 1997):

- drug distribution
- intracellular transport together with plasma levels
- mechanisms of drug metabolism and clearance
- tumour cell biochemistry
- the ability of the cell to repair damage and dose-limiting toxicity.

Clinical determinants and the use of chemotherapy

Traditionally, gastrointestinal cancers were treated with surgery alone, but chemotherapy is being increasingly used as a result of improved outcomes and quality of life in certain cancers. The decision to treat with chemotherapy is based on:

- site of the disease
- histology of the tumour
- stage of disease and size of tumour at presentation
- performance status of the patient
- aim of treatment, i.e. to cure, to prolong disease-free survival, or to palliate symptoms.

Chemotherapy can be used at various stages in the treatment of gastrointestinal cancers. It is used together with surgery or radiotherapy in a neoadjuvant setting or as an adjuvant, or it may be administered alone in a palliative setting, described below.

Neoadjuvant chemotherapy

Chemotherapy is administered before surgery with the aim of reducing the size of the tumour. The resultant tumour reduction increases the patient's eligibility for potentially curative surgery.

Adjuvant chemotherapy

Chemotherapy is given after primary treatment and is aimed at clinically undetectable disease for patients who have a high risk of recurrence.

Palliative chemotherapy

When a cure is not possible, chemotherapy may still be given to provide symptom control and to increase survival time.

The role of chemotherapy in the treatment of gastrointestinal cancers

Oesophageal and gastric cancer

Chemotherapy has proven efficacy in the treatment of oesphagogastric cancers. The most useful reported chemotherapy agents are cisplatin, protracted infusion 5FU, mitomycin C, methotrexate and paclitaxel, with cisplatin having the best response rate (Herskovic and Al-Sarraf, 1997). Epirubicin, cisplatin and 5FU (ECF) is a widely used regimen as it was found to have improved survival and quality of life advantages over 5FU, Doxorubcin and Methotrexate (FAMTX) (Webb et al., 1997). Trials are presently examining the role of taxanes, including docetaxel, the topoisomerase I inhibitor, irinotecan, oral fluoropyrimidines and Oxaliplatin.

Standard treatment for oesophageal cancer has traditionally been surgery and/or radiotherapy. Indeed surgery remains the optimal choice in early stage disease. However, it is of less value for most patients who present at an advanced stage, with only approximately 5% of these being cured (Ross et al., 1998).

Neoadjuvant chemotherapy for oesophageal cancer can be useful in downstaging the disease to aid surgical removal, enhance local control and eradicate microscopic disease. However, only 50% of patients will respond to the current available regimens (Roth et al., 1997). Recent evidence supports a multimodality approach with combination chemoradiation, using cisplatin and protracted venous infusion (PVI) 5FU. Cisplatin and 5FU have been demonstrated to act as radiosensitizers. A study by Al-Sarraf et al. (1997) demonstrated an improved median survival with chemoradiation for locally advanced tumours of 14.1 months, with 27% of patients achieving 5-year survival, against 9.3 months for radiotherapy alone with no survivors at 5 years. This is also supported by a small study by Meluch et al. (1997), where a 69% complete response was shown in patients receiving chemoradiation, using paclitaxel, carboplatin and protracted infusion 5FU. However, the use of adjuvant chemotherapy has not been proven.

Of patients with gastric cancer, 80% present with locally advanced or metastatic disease, resulting in a similar poor 5-year survival rate of 5–10% (Ross et al., 1998). A recent study (Webb et al., 1997) comparing combination therapies of epirubicin, cisplatin and protracted infusion 5FU (ECF) with 5FU, folinic acid, doxorubicin (Adriamycin) and methotrexate (FAMTX) demonstrated that patients receiving ECF obtained a 45% response rate with an overall survival of 8.9 months versus a 21% response and 5.7-month survival. Moreover, patients receiving the ECF arm reported an improved quality of life at 24 weeks. This regimen was proven useful in both primary gastric and oesophageal sites. Early trials using combination chemotherapy, in the neoadjuvant setting for advanced gastric cancer, have also shown good results (Cassidy, 1999). The development of agents interrupting the signalling pathways of cellular mechanisms that regulate cell growth look like promising treatments. Agents inhibiting epidermal growth factor receptor (EGFR), expressed on many human tissues are thought to be a trigger for the cellular growth mechanism (Yarden, 1988). Monoclonal antibodies directed against EGFR have been generated and are being investigated. The role of adjuvant chemotherapy is being investigated in national clinical trials.

Hepatic and biliary cancer

Hepatic and biliary cancers are very rare forms. Less than a third of patients presenting with biliary cancer are suitable for surgery at the time of diagnosis. National trials are currently examining the role of chemotherapy in the adjuvant setting. For inoperable or metastatic tumours, chemotherapy has been shown to provide symptomatic relief, for pain and jaundice, with some benefit in survival times. Glimelus et al. (1996) examined the use of 5FU, folinic acid (leucovorin) and etoposide (FELv) versus 5FU and folinic acid (FLv) versus best supportive care. The results demonstrated an increased survival time to 6 months versus 2.5 months.

Systemic chemotherapy for unresectable or metastatic hepatoma has not been very successful, providing only transient survival benefits. The most promising treatments include transarterial oily chemoembolization (TOCE) and percutaneous ethanol injection therapy (PEIT) for locally advanced adult liver cancer, although no standard treatment regimens have yet been established (Tempero and Rasmussen, 1996).

Pancreatic cancer

Cancer of the pancreas is a very aggressive disease. Complete surgical excision is the patient's best chance of survival, but this is associated with significant mortality and morbidity. Most patients present with advanced disease and their overall survival rate is less than 1% at 5 years, with most patients dying within the first year.

Adjuvant chemotherapy alone or combined with radiotherapy remains controversial (Ross et al., 1998). One randomized adjuvant study by Bakkevold et al. (1993) demonstrated an increased median survival from 11 months to 23 months, using six cycles of 5FU, doxorubicin and mitomycin C (FAM). However, there was no significant 5-year survival benefit. This regimen was not well tolerated and there were significant difficulties in recruiting patients. A European study for pancreatic cancer (ESPAC) has demonstrated a strong suggestion that adjuvant chemotherapy, 5FU or Gemcitabine, might be of benefit (Neoptolemos et al., 2002) and further studies are taking place. Results of further clinical trials are awaited. Neoadjuvant and adjuvant therapies are in their early stages and should be used only within the framework of clinical trials (Ross and Cunningham, 1999).

The use of palliative chemotherapy in advanced cases has been reported to improve the patient's quality of life and has some survival benefit. Gemcitabine or 5FU have been the most widely studied chemotherapeutic agent used for this disease and is one of the recommended standard treatments. Protracted infusion 5FU used in phase II clinical trials demonstrated a 15–20% response rate (Hidalgo et al., 1999). A combination of cisplatin and protracted infusion 5FU was shown to improve the performance status for 34% of patients and provide significant symptom control, but no significant survival benefits (Nicolson et al., 1995). Gemcitabine was compared with bolus 5FU. The results showed an improvement in pain and performance status of 23% for gemcitabine and 4.8% for 5FU and 1-year survival rates of 18% versus 2% (Burris et al., 1997). However, there is some controversy over how 5FU is administered and how it is selected. A 30-minute infusion of 5FU has been shown to be of suboptimal efficacy against a bolus injection (Ross and Cunningham, 1999).

For the future a possible new agent may include a cholecystokinin and gastrin receptor antagonist. These hormones are thought to encourage growth in pancreatic cancer.

Colorectal cancer

Surgery continues to play the major role in the treatment and cure of colon cancer. However, of the 75% of colorectal cancer patients who receive curative surgery, half will undergo a recurrence. The recurrence rate is dependent on the stage of disease noted at surgery. The 5-year survival rate for Dukes' A stage carcinoma is 80%, for Dukes' B 65% and for Dukes' C 30% (Sumpter and Cunningham, 1998). For patients with unresectable liver metastases, a recent review of the literature indicated that the disease might be successfully downstaged for surgery using combination chemotherapy regimens. This approach has resulted in a 40% 5-year survival rate in this group of patients (Groeghan and Scheele, 1999).

Adjuvant chemotherapy for Dukes' C patients has shown benefit in terms of a 15% increase in survival rates against surgery alone (Ross and Cunningham, 1999). 5FU is the accepted standard agent used for the treatment of colorectal cancer and several infusion regimens are now available. A study carried out by the North Central Cancer Treatment Group (NCCTG) comparing observation with the administration of adjuvant 5FU, folinic acid, given as a bolus on days 1–5 every 4–6 weeks, has shown, after 6 years, an improvement in time to relapse and survival rates for Dukes' C patients (O'Connell et al., 1997). The inclusion of folinic acid potentiates the action of

5FU. A further study comparing PVI 5FU with consecutive 5-day boluses of 5FU (NCCTG) demonstrated a significant reduction in toxicity for a similar patient group (Ross and Cunningham, 1999).

For Dukes' B patients the results are not quite so clear. A pooled analysis of five randomized trials, by Erhlichman et al. (1997), demonstrated survival benefits of 81–83%. Further studies are presently being carried out. In the light of the current data, Ross and Cunningham (1999) suggest that adjuvant systemic treatment be offered to stage B2 and B3 patients using careful patient selection based on individual clinical and performance status basis. National clinical trials are now assessing the value of combination chemotherapy in the adjuvant setting.

Randomized trials have established the role of palliative chemotherapy. Scheithauer et al. (1993) illustrated an increase in survival from 5 months to 11 months when patients received a chemotherapy regimen including systemic 5FU, compared with best supportive care. However, no one 5FU regimen has been unanimously accepted as the 'gold' standard and several different regimens are used. A 48-hour 2-weekly regimen, comprising a 2-hour infusion of folinic acid, bolus 5FU, and a 22-hour infusion of 5FU for 2 consecutive days, was shown to have greater response rates than the NCCTG regimen (DeGramont et al., 1997). Phase III clinical trials have now been completed which compare an oral fluoropyrimidine (Capecitabine) to bolus 5FU in patients with advanced colorectal cancer (Hoff, 2000). These trials demonstrated a superior tumour response rate for Capecitabine with an equivalent overall survival rate (Van Cutsem, 2001). Examples of 5FU administration include:

- PVI 5FU
- 48-hour weekly 5FU alone or with oral folinic acid
- 48-hour 2-weekly 5FU and folinic acid
- 24-hour weekly high-dose 5FU
- oral preparation of 5FU (recently received UK licence).

The addition of mitomycin C to protracted infusion 5FU demonstrated a 54% versus 38% response rate, with an improvement in failure-free survival, although it was shown to have no overall survival benefit (Ross et al., 1997). Most recent studies have shown that irinotecan (CPT II) is a valuable option as second-line treatment for 5FU-resistant disease in patients who maintain a good performance status (Cunningham et al., 1997–8). Further studies are now examining the combination of irinotecan to 48-hour bimonthly and weekly 24-hour high-dose 5FU regimens in first-line treatment (Ross and Cunningham, 1999).

New drugs include oxaliplatin and raltitrexed, both of which provide further treatment options for this patient group (Kohne, 1999). Saltz et al. (2001) have also shown that a monoclonal antibody (Cetuximab), an agent inhibiting the molecular signalling pathway regulating cell growth, is active in colorectal cancer. Immunization with CEA Vaccine (CEAVAC), a molecule that stimulates the body's own immune defence mechanisms, is also being evaluated.

Rectal cancer

Rectal cancer has a recurrence rate of 25–30% after complete resection. Clinical trials have indicated that adjuvant chemotherapy improves survival for patients with stage II and III disease (Labianca, 1999). Recurrence rates were reduced to 41.5% with adjuvant chemoradiation compared with 62.7% with radiotherapy alone (Krook et al., 1991).

Recent advances in staging techniques have now made it possible to select high-risk patients for neoadjuvant chemotherapy (Taylor et al., 1999). Chemoradiation, using PVI 5FU and mitomycin C may be of greater advantage preoperatively, giving the advantage of sphincter preservation and increased resectability rates in locally advanced disease (Labianca, 1999). With the advent of new drugs, with proven efficacy for the treatment of colorectal cancer, trials are investigating the value of combination oral 5FU (Capecitabine) and Oxalipatin together with radiotherapy in the treatment of rectal cancer.

The nursing role and the patient's experience

Nurses are very likely to meet patients diagnosed with gastrointestinal cancer as a quarter of cancers diagnosed in England and Wales are of this nature. To provide effective clinical care it is important that nurses have specialist knowledge and skills. To be effective, they need to be capable of accurate assessment, diagnosis and intervention (Jenkins, 1996). Knowledge should include an understanding of the nature and effects of gastrointestinal cancers, and skills should include competence in the administration and management of chemotherapy and its side effects. The ability to communicate effectively and a positive relationship with the patient are essential components of the delivery of care.

Patients with gastrointestinal cancers undergo changes to their 'basic' everyday life. Their digestive system is disturbed, causing difficulty with eating, weight loss, diarrhoea or constipation. This, in turn, causes barriers in socialization with friends and family and often leads to an altered body image and embarrassment, particularly when having to discuss topics such as bowel habits. Nurses must constantly help patients to meet the challenges of everyday living interrupted and altered by disease and treatment (Holmes, 1990a). To communicate and help effectively the nurse must gain the patient's trust. To gain trust, good working relationships need to be formed between patients and nurses. Benner (1984) showed that such relationships can positively affect patients' progress by enhancing a climate of support, patient involvement and control.

Specifically, nurses can influence patients' experience of chemotherapy, which plays a significant role in treatment. The idea of receiving chemotherapy is often frightening and many patients have preconceived beliefs. Therefore, nursing care needs to encompass both the physical and psychological aspects. The reduced socialization that the patient may already be experiencing may be enhanced by general weakness, inability to concentrate or hair loss, all induced by chemotherapy. This isolation may bring about feelings of despair and also impact on close family relationships (Holmes, 1985). Therefore, provision of accurate information about methods of administration and treatment, and effective care of side effects, will help to reduce the patient's and the family's anxiety. Prompt diagnosis and intervention, by the nurse, for chemotherapy-induced side effects can provide considerable relief to distress (Tanghe et al., 1998). However, the management of side effects often requires a team effort, involving family, friends and the community nursing team because some side effects will occur when the patient is at home. The dissemination of information and education to relevant people and professionals is an essential part of care. It is tempting to provide masses of information, but it should be remembered that optimum care can be achieved only if each patient's unique situation is taken into account (Holmes, 1990a and b). Information giving should be tailored to suit the individual.

The ability to provide such care grows as the nurse becomes an expert in his or her field.

On completion of chemotherapy, the patient is generally relieved; however, some patients become insecure and afraid. They no longer have the security of regular hospital visits and the infusion of drugs treating their cancer. Continuity of care through a follow-up management plan is important.

Nursing care of intravenous devices and the handling of chemotherapy

Handling and administering chemotherapy

Cytotoxic agents need to be handled carefully because they are known to be carcinogenic, fetotoxic and genotoxic. Exposure to these risks occurs during preparation, administration and disposal (Bean, 1996). Many cytotoxic agents are irritant to soft tissue and some are capable of causing necrosis; these are called vesicants (Mallett and Dougherty, 2000). Therefore, great care should be taken to avoid skin contamination or inadvertent infusion of the agent into cellular tissue (extravasation). Patients handling their own chemotherapy, e.g. 5FU infusions, must also be informed of appropriate precautions. The care required when administering chemotherapy peripherally is illustrated in the Table 9.1.

The correct disposal of cytotoxic agents, syringes and infusion bags is also crucial. These should be disposed of in a labelled, sealed and water-tight container, which must then be taken to one of the specific sites at the hospital or local surgery for appropriate destruction (Bean, 1996). Patients with 5FU infusions at home must be given the appropriate instruction and equipment for correct and safe disposal.

Routes of administration

There are now a number of intravenous devices and routes through which patients may receive their chemotherapy, e.g. via peripheral cannulas, centrally placed skin-tunnelled catheters (STCs) or peripherally inserted central catheters (PICCs). These are explained briefly.

Peripheral cannulas

Placing the cannulas safely and effectively requires specialist training and practice (Mallett and Dougherty, 2000). The care of

Table 9.1 Care of peripheral intravenous administration of cytotoxic agents

Action	Rationale
Explanation of procedure to patient	To gain the patients verbal/written consent
Gloves and apron worn	Prevent contamination of the practitioner
Prepare equipment needed for aseptic intravenous administration	Prevent infection
Check infusion, syringe label against prescription chart and patient identification at bedside	To ensure correct dose given to correct patient
Check intravenous device site is satisfactory and patency of the vein	To detect phlebitis and displacement of cannula
Ensure rate of infusion is correct and be aware of potential adverse effects	To avoid speed shock and overloading; to be able to manage immediate side effects
Administer vesicant agents first	Give most potentially tissue-damaging drugs when venous integrity is at its best
Observe vein throughout bolus injection and regularly during infusions	Be able to recognize early signs and symptoms of extravasation to minimize adverse effect
Check patient's comfort throughout	Reduce patient distress
Record administration on prescription chart	Prevent duplication of treatment and as a record of treatment

Adapted from Mallet and Dougherty (2000).

peripheral cannulas should include: ensured patency, sterile, comfortable dressings, regular inspection of the insertion site, and the ability to recognize signs of complications (Dougherty, 1997).

Skin-tunnelled catheters and peripherally inserted central catheters

Administration of chemotherapy via an STC or a PICC is performed for the following reasons: poor general peripheral venous access, patient's needle phobia, administration of a protracted venous infusion or convenience to reduce the patient's hospital stay.

An STC is usually inserted into the chest wall, tunnelled under the skin to the shoulder, where it is inserted into the subclavian or axillary vein; it then proceeds until the tip is positioned in the right atrium. A PICC is inserted directly into the vein in the antecubital fossa and ends in the distal third of the superior vena cava (Berg, 1996).

Care of intravenous sites

Infections are commonly caused by *Staphylococcus epidermidis* or other skin flora, taking care of the exit sites is therefore of paramount importance. Cleansing of the exit site and upper incision with 0.5% chlorhexidine in 70% alcohol is the recommended method (Harrison, 1997).

Patients with STCs can allow the exit site to get wet in a shower; the PICC exit site needs to be kept dry because the catheter is directly inserted to the vein. A review by Cook (1999) suggests that the optimum, cost-effective dressing is a transparent (TSP) dressing, such as Opsite 3000, applied 24 hours after catheter insertion and changed every 5–7 days. Alternatively, patients with STCs who are unable to apply transparent dressings effectively may use sterile dry gauze changed daily. PICCs need to be secured well and held in place with a bandage to minimize the risk of catching the extension set on clothing. Regular inspection of the insertion site for complications is essential (Dougherty, 1997)

Patency of lumina

Lumina used for intermittent therapy must be flushed after each use and at least once a week if not accessed within that time (Mallett and Dougherty, 2000). Suggested flushing solution is 0.9% sodium chloride if the catheter is used intermittently every day or heparinized saline (50 units of heparin in 5 ml 0.9% saline) if the lumen is unused for 7 days (Mallett and Dougherty, 2000). Recommended flushing techniques include employing a push-pause method of solution instillation and the maintenance of a positive pressure when clamping closed the lumen. Table 9.2 illustrates the care of possible complications

Nursing management of chemotherapy-induced side effects

Stomatitis

Stomatitis is caused by damage to the mucous membrane of the oral cavity and about 40% of patients receiving chemotherapy suffer from this side effect. It is one of the most common side

Table 9.2 Complications associated with central venous access devices: recognition and actions

Complication	Signs and symptoms	Action
Local skin infection	Redness, swelling, tenderness or purulent discharge from exit site	Swab; refer to doctor; oral or intravenous antibiotics
In PICCs hlebitis (mechanical) usually occurs with 24–48 hours or within 1 week of insertion	As above – occurring at the insertion site or along the route of a PICC	Apply warmth to the area. Evaluate over next 72 hours; if not resolved remove catheter
Systemic infection	Fever (≥38°C) or rigors May be associated with flushing of the catheter	Take blood cultures – centrally from catheter and peripherally Refer to doctor for intravenous antibiotics and possible removal of catheter
Superior vena cava, subclavian or axillary vein thrombosis (anywhere along the catheter)	Pain, generalized swelling, redness and warmth in associated shoulder, neck or arm	Refer to doctor for Doppler ultrasonography to confirm diagnosis. Anticoagulation therapy and removal of catheter
Displacement of or break in catheter	Discomfort, localized swelling and/or difficulties with infusion/flushing	Refer to doctor x-ray check Check catheter integrity on radiograph using radiosensitive dye
Occlusion of catheter lumen	Difficulty flushing catheter	Instillation of fibrinolytic agent for 2 hours and then withdrawal of blood

effects for patients receiving chemotherapy for gastrointestinal cancers. The cells in the oral cavity undergo a 7- to 10-day cycle of renewal and are thus susceptible to damage from chemotherapy (Lembersky and Posner, 1996). This inflammatory reaction may progress to painful ulceration and secondary infection, although in the early stages the patient may complain of tenderness presenting with mild erythema (Holmes, 1996). Drugs that commonly cause stomatitis include anti-metabolites such as 5FU and methotrexate, and antibiotics, such as doxorubicin, by interfering with cell renewal via the inhibition of cell division of the basal layer (Miller, 1998). Epithelial hyperplasia or dysplasia and collagen and glandular degeneration may also occur as a result of chemotherapy (Berger and Kilroy, 1997).

Although it may not be possible to prevent stomatitis from occurring, early detection and good oral hygiene can minimize the risk of secondary systemic infection and reduce further discomfort to the patient. A widely used assessment tool was developed by the World Health Organization (WHO, 1997). This tool describes and grades the severity of stomatitis and acts as a guide for practitioners, particularly for prescribing appropriate care (Table 9.3).

Table 9.3 International toxicity guidelines – stomatitis

Grade	0	1	2	3	4
Stomatitis	None	Painless ulcers, erythema or mild soreness in the absence of lesions	Painful erythema, oedema or ulcers, but can eat or swallow	Painful erythema, oedema or ulcers Difficulty taking fluids/ solids orally	Severe ulceration or requires parenteral or enteral nutritional support

Good general oral hygiene should be encouraged by a suggested daily routine. This should be discussed with the patient in order to increase the patient's understanding and compliance. The mouth should be rinsed and the teeth should be brushed, using a soft toothbrush, after every meal and at bedtime, removing any food substances left behind (Holmes, 1996). Dentures should also be removed and cleaned each time. There is some debate over the type of mouthwash to be recommended, although it is agreed that it should not contain alcohol, because this dries the mucosa. However, the importance of the frequency and consistency of practice is paramount (Wilkes, 1996). Chlorhexidine gluconate 0.12% 10–15 ml diluted in a tumbler of water has been shown to have some broad-spectrum antimicrobial activity and beneficial prophylactic benefits in bone marrow transplant recipients, but has not been proven in chemotherapy outpatients (Miller, 1998).

Prophylactic use of ice chips held in the patient's mouth for 30 minutes, 5 minutes before chemotherapy administration, is suggested to reduce stomatitis for bolus administration of 5FU (Mahood et al., 1991). However, this technique is not always easily tolerated by patients and further studies dispute its preventive effects. Once stomatitis has occurred, the use of sucralfate emulsion, rinsed around the mouth four times a day, may give some protection and beneficial stimulation to the inflamed mucosa. The patient must not take anything orally for 10–15 minutes after this treatment, allowing the solution to have maximum contact with the eroded areas (Loprinzi et al., 1997). If acute stomatitis has occurred (grade 3–4 described above), continuous infusions of 5FU must be discontinued to allow the patient to recover. In severe cases the patient may require hospitalization. Analgesia may be necessary to relieve pain and to enable the patient to take an oral diet.

Diarrhoea

The epithelium cells of the intestines have a rapid turnover rate and are damaged by chemotherapy, particularly anti-metabolites. The mucosal cells become ulcerated and inflamed and produce increased amounts of mucus, the peristaltic rate is increased and the result is an increased throughput of intestinal substances (Wilkes, 1996). In severe cases of diarrhoea the patient may become dehydrated, hypotensive or suffer from a related neutropenic sepsis if the granulocyte nadir occurs at the same time (Allegra and Grem, 1997). This can be debilitating, exhausting and very upsetting for the patient. It is important therefore that even the mildest diarrhoea is reported and controlled. Nutritional management by encouraging the patient to take adequate fluids, proteins and calories is an important nursing intervention (Wilkes, 1996). Pharmacological management is also often necessary and may include such drugs as loperamide, a long-acting opiate, which reduces ileal calcium fluxes, or codeine, which reduces secretions and peristalsis and is much more constipating than morphine (Linn, 1998). If diarrhoea is persistent, it may be necessary to discontinue, delay or reduce the dose of the contributory chemotherapy agent. Fluorouracil, irinotecan, doxorubicin and methotrexate, all of which may be used for the treatment of gastrointestinal cancers, have a high propensity to cause diarrhoea. The WHO (1997) common toxicity criteria include an assessment tool for grading the severity of diarrhoea (Table 9.4).

Palmar–plantar erythema (hand–foot syndrome)

This side effect may also be a dose-limiting factor and, although it is only related to FU toxicity, it is well worth mentioning. This syndrome tends to occur mostly with the protracted infusions of

Table 9.4 International toxicity guidelines – diarrhoea

Grade	0	1	2	3	4
Diarrhoea	None	Increase of less than four stools/ day over pretreatment	Increase of four to six stools/day or nocturnal stools	Increase of more than seven stools/ day or incontinence, or need for parenteral support for dehydration	Physiological consequences requiring intensive care

5FU (Allegra and Grem, 1997). Redness on the palms of the hands or soles of the feet occur, followed by a dryness and cracking of the skin which is often accompanied by tenderness and tingling. This can be severe enough to limit the patient's dexterity and/or mobility. Early detection and the prescription of vitamin B$_6$ tablets may control this effect. However, if the syndrome is severe, the chemotherapy will be discontinued or delayed and the dose reduced to avoid recurrence (Table 9.5).

Table 9.5 International toxicity guidelines – palmar–plantar erythema

Grade	0	1	2	3	4
Palmar–plantar erythema	None	Skin changes or dermatitis without pain (e.g. erythema, peeling)	Skin changes with pain, not interfering with function	Skin changes with pain, interfering with function	

Fatigue

Fatigue is a common side effect induced by chemotherapy. The physiological mechanism of this debilitating side effect is unknown. There is no definitive description of what fatigue is because it is a subjective personal experience, which affects mental and bodily functions (Portenoy and Miaskowski, 1998). Fatigue can be debilitating and have a widespread effect on everyday activities resulting in a negative effect on psychological well-being (Winningham, 1996). Patients receiving protracted infusion of 5FU and mitomycin C, or combination chemotherapy, appear to suffer from this side effect to varying degrees.

Management of fatigue is dependent on a comprehensive assessment of the patient's own symptoms and other contributory factors. Effective interventions often follow a trial-and-error regimen to find the best solution. Alteration in nutrition, daily activities, rest patterns, exercise, stress management, correction of anaemia and patient education may minimize the effects of fatigue (Portenoy and Miaskowski, 1998).

Nausea and vomiting

Nausea and vomiting are well documented as being one of the most distressing side effects of chemotherapy as perceived by patients. Nurses are in an ideal position to improve the management and negative impact of chemotherapy by improving symptom control (Johnson et al., 1997). Although the way in which chemotherapy induces nausea and vomiting is not fully understood, the mechanism of emesis is known and new pharmacological agents have been discovered. One of the major advances has been the advent of the serotonin (5HT) antagonists (Hogan, 1997).

Receptors, which may be hormones, growth factors or neurotransmitters, located on cells bind to or are activated by messenger molecules, which result in the commencement of the vomiting reflex (Hawthorn et al., 1991). Once receptors, largely found in the gastrointestinal tract or liver, have been stimulated by toxins, a message is sent to an area known as the chemoreceptor zone in the area postrema of the brain and from there to another area called the vomiting centre located within the brain stem. The vomiting centre then brings about the action of vomiting. Other pathways include the impact of emotion and sight on the higher brain centres of the cortex and limbic systems, resulting in anticipatory vomiting or effects on the sympathetic nervous system from distension or irritation of the gastrointestinal tract, kidneys or bladder (Wilkes, 1996).

Nausea and vomiting may be described as acute, i.e. occurring within 24 hours of treatment, or delayed, i.e. after the first 24 hours. Cisplatin, doxorubicin and methotrexate usually cause emesis within 1–3 hours of treatment, but with carboplatin emesis may occur 12–18 hours later; delayed emesis may also be caused by cisplatin and tends to be dose related (Pisters and Kris, 1998). The use of oral dexamethasone is thought to inhibit prostaglandin release and thus interrupt the stimulus to vomit. This, together with oral metoclopramide, a 5HT, and dopamine antagonist, has been shown to be more effective in combination than alone. However, the combination of a serotonin antagonist and a corticosteriod has been shown to be the most effective prophylaxis so far and is recommended as a standard prophylactic antiemetic treatment (Pisters and Kris, 1998).

Alopecia

Hair loss can have an impact on a patient's quality of life, altering body image and having a negative effect on self-esteem (Howser, 1996). Alopecia acts as a reminder to patients that they have cancer and informs others that they are not well, and it can lead to depression and humiliation (Chernecky, 1998). Anti-metabolites, alkylating agents and antibiotics may all cause alopecia to a lesser or greater degree (Wilkes, 1996). The amount of hair loss and the time before regrowth is dependent on the dose and duration of treatment (Wilkes, 1996). Hair loss can occur as early as 2 weeks after the first treatment, and it may be rapid and lead to complete loss. Chemotherapy-induced hair loss is usually temporary; however, on regrowth hair may change in texture and colour, and may be curlier (Seipp, 1998). Preparation of the patient for this is important; professional help should be provided and the patient should be offered a wig or head scarf (Howser, 1996). A hair-preservation technique that involves causing peripheral vasoconstriction by scalp cooling may be offered to patients receiving bolus doses, or short infusions, of chemotherapy. This has shown to be more effective with single-agent chemotherapy than with combination chemotherapy (Chernecky, 1998). Other practical interventions to minimize hair loss should be suggested: avoidance, if possible, of the use of hot hair dryers, electric hair curlers, hair spray or dyes. Ideally, the hair should be left in a natural state, left to dry without aid after washing and generally treated in a gentle manner when grooming (Chernecky, 1998).

Bone marrow suppression

Bone marrow suppression, although usually transient, is the key dose-limiting side effect of many chemotherapy agents because the haemopoietic system is a highly active organ of cell regeneration and is susceptible to therapy-related cell destruction (Jakubowski, 1996). The degree of bone marrow suppression is related to the dose and duration of treatment. It can be split into three distinct areas: low haemoglobin leading to anaemia, reduction in white blood cells leading to septicaemia and a reduction of thrombocytes leading to haemorrhage.

Anaemia is a reduction of haemoglobin and erythrocytes which results in symptoms of tiredness and breathlessness, but can be resolved with a blood transfusion. A shortage of thrombocytes increases the risk of haemorrhage which may present obliquely as oral blood blisters, spontaneous bruising or as an obvious bleed. Platelet transfusions are available for gross thrombocytopenia or symptomatic patients. However, it is usually managed by waiting for a natural increment of thrombocytes before administering the next dose of chemotherapy. The risk of gastrointestinal bleeding in patients with primary tumours of the gastrointestinal tract may be increased by the administration of cytotoxic agents (Lembersky and Posner, 1996).

The increased susceptibility to infection as a result of a reduction of leucocytes, particularly the neutrophils, is a major area of concern that can lead to fatal results. Early detection of sepsis is imperative to avoid progression to septic shock. Clinical features include fever, chills, confusion, rapid pulse and respiration (Klemn and Hubbard, 1992). Generally the reduction in leucocytes (nadir) occurs from approximately day 5 post-treatment to day 14, with day 10 being the lowest point (Schafer, 1998). However, some drugs have a potential for longer nadir such as carboplatin. Risk factors include systemic infection arising from the oral cavity or from an ulcerated, irritated gastrointestinal tract, and if present from the STC or PICC.

Patient selection criteria

The medical criteria evaluating the stage of disease and the patient's general health status are the clinician's guiding factors when deciding appropriate treatment regimens (Garvey and Kramer, 1983). Strict clinical trial criteria dictate the eligibility of patient selection for various regimens. The selection criteria also include an assessment of the patient's psychological and physical status. Two commonly used physical assessment guides are illustrated in Table 9.6.

Patients chosen for protracted infusion regimens should be willing and able to participate in their own care or have a significant carer who will provide such care (Schulmeister, 1992). Other considerations to be taken into account are personal hygiene practices, home environment, psychosocial status, cognitive skills and physical abilities (Reville and Almadrones, 1989).

Table 9.6 Performance status scales

Karnofsky		Zubrod–ECOG–WHO	
Condition	Scale	Scale	Condition
Normal, no complaints	100	0	Normal activity
Able to carry out normal activity	90	1	Symptoms – normal activity
Cares for self Unable to carry on normal active work	70	2	Symptomatic, but in bed < 50% of the day
Requires considerable assistance and frequent medical care	50	3	Needs to be in bed > 50% of the day
Severely disabled Hospitalization indicated	30	4	Unable to get out of bed
Dead	0	5	Dead

Minna et al. (1984 – reduced version).
ECOG, European Co-operative Oncology Group;
WHO, World Health Organization.

The role of clinical trials

The purpose of clinical trials is to ascertain the effective dose of the drug, the optimum method of administration and the potential side effects, and to test the effectiveness of new regimens or drugs and improve on standard therapies (Simon, 1997).

Clinical trials are usually carried out over three phases, described below. The objectives of each trial must be clearly stated in a written protocol. The treatment plan, monitoring methods and other pharmaceutical guidelines should be identified to ensure good patient care (Jenkins, 1996).

1. Phase I trials aim to determine the optimal and safe dose of the drug and method of administration. Patients offered these trials usually have no effective therapeutic options and, as the study is to evaluate the dose and not the efficacy, patients with any type of cancer may be entered (Simon, 1997). Often fewer than 100 patients may receive the new treatment before it is tested in a phase II study.
2. Phase II trials look at the anti-tumour effect of a new agent or new combination of agents. Patients are entered who have a particular type of cancer or related cancers. There may be several trials, which involve hundreds of patients with many

types of selected cancers. The patients entered into these trials usually have measurable disease and are required to have a good performance status (Jenkins, 1996).

3. Phase III is when one or more treatments are compared against already proven standard treatments; these treatments may include new drugs or new combinations. These trials often look at various scenarios, e.g. disease-free survival, response rates, quality of life or pattern of recurrence. The results of phase III trials are the most likely to change clinical practice, e.g. the comparison of irinotecan versus best supportive care in advanced colorectal cancer (Cunningham et al., 1997–8).

Patient information/education

Effective provision of information and education to patients is a crucial area of care (Dougherty et al., 1998). Patients have to make many decisions during their treatment. With more treatment options and clinical trials available, and the changing tide of attitudes, patients are now active participants in their treatment management plans. Patients may have to make changes to their working life and find ways of adapting to their diagnosis and treatment regimens (Holmes, 1990a and b). However, well-informed patients can minimize and pave the way for these changes if they are provided with appropriate information. Also, as previously mentioned, complications while undergoing chemotherapy can be reduced, with early detection and treatment, by patient participation (Taplin et al., 1997). Patient participation in care has grown with the advent of PVI 5FU, via centrally placed catheters, and many patients are managed solely on an outpatient basis (Nightingale et al., 1996). Oral preparations of 5FU provide the patient with greater control over their treatment and avoid the distress related to the intravenous devices. However patients should be given clear written guidance on how and when to take their medication in order to avoid serious mistakes. A diary is a useful tool for the patient to record the occurrence of side effects, the dose and time to take the medication. If the patient is not seen regularly at clinic the set up of a 'telephone clinic' may be a useful way of monitoring patients well being.

Effective communication is difficult in the presence of a state of anxiety. Anxiety is well recognized in association with a diagnosis of cancer, the administration of chemotherapy and hospitalization (Payne and Massie, 1998).). This state of anxiety can lead to reduced ability to concentrate and an increased feeling of vulnerability (Clark, 1992). Leydon et al. (2000) suggest that, although all patients desire basic information about diagnosis and treatment, not all want greater detail. The researchers also suggest that further investigation is needed to ascertain when and how to provide information. Information provided effectively can return some control to the patient, which in turn reduces anxiety (Holmes, 1996).

Information promotes patient autonomy, arming patients with the necessary facts and enabling them to give their consent or otherwise for treatment. This is called 'informed consent' (Kodish et al., 1997). Patients must be 18 years or over and have decision-making capabilities (Emanuel, 1998). Suggested basic information should include understanding of:

- the diagnosis
- the nature, risks and benefits of the proposed intervention
- the alternative treatments
- the likely results of no treatment
- the likelihood of success.

(Shapiro, 1998).

A structured, well-planned, teaching programme has been shown to benefit the patient (Lowry, 1995). This, given on a one-to-one basis, allows flexibility to take into account patients' individual needs and abilities (Dougherty et al., 1997, 1998). Effective education is crucial for the successful completion of any treatment. The patient and family must acquire skills and knowledge about the drugs and equipment (Chrystal, 1997). Practical demonstrations, where necessary, and written handouts increase the effectiveness of the teaching programme (Butler, 1984). A study by Whitman-Obhert (1996) showed that patients and families were appreciative of concise, easily understood, written handouts. Teaching and written information should be comprehensive

To optimize learning, the time and environment for teaching need to be carefully selected and reinforced during the patient's admission. The amount of self-care taken on by the patient and amount of support required from the community nurse should form discussions between the nurse and patient (Dougherty et al., 1997, 1998). Therefore, it is crucial to set up support from the community nurse and GP before the patient's discharge. Ongoing support for patients receiving protracted infusions of chemotherapy is essential (Dougherty et al., 1997, 1998).

Conclusions

The importance of the specialist nurse has been identified and acknowledged. It is not just skill and knowledge that are valuable. The caring professional relationship formed between the patient and the nurse can enhance the person's ability to cope with difficult treatments.

Knowledge of the cell cycle, drug mechanisms and the purpose of clinical trials provides the necessary theoretical background. This, together with an awareness of the current regimens used for the treatment of gastrointestinal cancers, is essential to providing good nursing care. Careful consideration must be given to the appropriate and safe administration of cytotoxic drugs, symptom control, patient education and information, maintenance of patient independence and care of the family. The specialist-trained nurse needs to apply his or her skills and knowledge in an individual manner appropriate to the patient.

Treatments for gastrointestinal cancer are continually being advanced. Regimens and methods of administration are managed to obtain optimal advantage. It is the responsibility of the specialist nurse to keep up to date with changing treatments and practice in order to provide excellent quality patient care.

References

Ahlgren J (1992) Principles of chemotherapy in gastrointestinal cancer. In: Ahlgren J, Macdonald J (eds), Gastrointestinal Oncology. Philadelphia, PA: Lippincott & Co.

Allegra C, Grem J (1997) Antimetabolites. In: DeVita V, Hellman S, Rosenberg S (eds), Cancer Principles and Practice of Oncology, 5th edn. Philadelphia, PA: Lippincott-Raven.

Al-Sarraf M, Martz K, Herkovic A et al. (1997) Progress report of combined chemoradiotherapy versus radiotherapy alone in patients with oesophageal cancer: an intergroup study. Journal of Clinical Oncology 15: 277-284.

Bakkevold K, Arnesjo B, Dahl O, Kambestad B (1993) Adjuvant combination chemotherapy (AMF) following radical resection of carcinoma of the pancreas and ampulla of Vater - results of a controlled, prospective randomised multi-centre study. European Journal of Cancer 29A: 698-703.

Bean C (1996) The safe handling of cancer chemotherapeutic agents. In: DeVita V, Hellman S, Rosenberg S (eds), Cancer Principles and Practice of Oncology, 5th edn. Philadelphia, PA: Lippincott-Raven.

Beck W, Dalton W (1997) Pharmacology of cancer chemotherapy - mechanisms of drug resistance In: DeVita V, Hellman S, Rosenberg S (eds), Cancer Principles and Practice of Oncology, 5th edn. Philadelphia, PA: Lippincott-Raven.

Benner P (1984) The helping role. In: From Novice to Expert, Vol 4. CA: Addison-Wesley, pp. 47-75.

Berg D (1996) Drug delivery systems. In: Burke MB, Wilkes GM, Ingwersen K, Bean C, Berg D (eds), Cancer Chemotherapy: A nursing process approach, 2nd edn. Boston, MA: Jones & Bartlett.

Berger A, Kilroy T (1997) Oral complications. In: DeVita V, Hellman S, Rosenberg S (eds), Cancer Principles and Practice of Oncology, 5th edn. Philadelphia, PA: Lippincott-Raven.

Burris III H, Moore M, Andersen J et al. (1997) Improvements in survival and clinical benefit with gemcitabine as first line therapy for patients with advanced pancreas cancer: a randomized trial. Journal of Clinical Oncology 15: 2403-2413.

Butler M (1984) Families response to chemotherapy by an ambulatory infusion pump. Nursing Clinics of North America 19: 139-143.

Cassidy J (1999) Stomach. Gastrointestinal Cancer. International reviews of clinical developments in gastrointestinal cancers. Rhone-Poulenc Rorer.

Chernecky C (1998) Alopecia. In: Yasko J (ed.), Nursing Management of Symptoms Associated with Chemotherapy, 4th edn. Bala Cynwyd, PA: Meniscus Health Care Communications.

Chrystal C (1997) Administering continuous vesicant chemotherapy in the ambulatory setting. Journal of Intravenous Nursing 20: 78-88.

Clark J (1992) Psychosocial dimensions: The patient. In: Groenwald S, Frogge M, Goodman M, Yarbo C (eds), Psychosocial Dimensions of Cancer. Boston, MA: Jones & Bartlett.

Cook N (1999) Central venous catheters: preventing infection and occlusion. British Journal of Nursing 3: 981-988.

Cunningham D, Pyrhonen S, James R et al. (1997-8): A phase III multicentre randomized study of cpt ii versus supportive care alone in patients with 5FU resistant metastatic colorectal cancer. The Lancet 352: 1413-1418.

DeGramont A, Bosset J-F, Milan C et al. (1997) Randomised trial comparing monthly low-dose leucovorin and fluorouracil bolus with bimonthly high-dose leucovorin and fluorouracil bolus plus continuous infusion for advanced colorectal cancer: a French Intergroup study. Journal of Clinical Oncology 15: 808-815.

Dougherty L (1997) Reducing the risk of complications in IV therapy. Nursing Standard 12. 5: 40-42.

Dougherty L, Viner C, Young J (1998): Establishing ambulatory chemotherapy at home. Professional Nurse 13.6: 356-358.

Emanuel L (1998) Advance directives. In: Berger A, Portenoy R, Weissman D (eds), Principles and Practice of Supportive Oncology. Philadelphia, PA: Lippincott-Raven.

Erhlichman C, Marsoni S, Seitz J et al. (1997) Event free and overall survival is increased by FUFA in resected b colon cancer; a pooled analysis of 5 randomised controlled trials (RCT). Proceedings of the American Society of Clinical Oncology 16: 991.

Garvey E, Kramer R (1983) Improving cancer patients adjustments to infusion chemotherapy: Evaluation of a patient education program. Cancer Nursing Oct: 373-378.

Glimelius B, Hoffman K, Sjoden P-O et al. (1996) Chemotherapy improves survival and quality of life in advanced pancreatic and biliary cancer. Annals of Oncology 5: 593-600.

Groeghan J, Scheele J (1999) The treatment of colorectal liver metastases. British Journal of Surgery 86: 158–169.

Harrison M (1997) Central venous catheters: a review of the literature. Nursing Standard 11.27: 43–45.

Hawthorn J, Tiffany R, Pritchard P et al. (1991) The physiology of nausea and vomiting. In: The Management of Nausea and Vomiting Induced by Chemotherapy and Radiotherapy, Vol 2. Glaxo Holdings plc, pp. 19–49.

Herskovic A, Al-Sarraf M (1997) Combination of 5-fluorouracil and radiation in oesophageal cancer. Seminars in Radiation Oncology 7: 283–290.

Hidalgo M, Castellano D, Paz-Ares L et al. (1999) Phase I–II study of gemcitabine and fluorouracil as a continuous infusion in patients with pancreatic cancer. Journal of Clinical Oncology 17: 585–592.

Hoff PM (2000) Capecitabine as first-line treatment for colorectal cancer (CRC): integrated results of 1207 patients (pts) from 2 randomised, phase III studies. On behalf of the Capecitabine CRC Study Group. Annals of Oncology 11 (supplement 4): 60a.

Hogan C (1997) Cancer nursing: the art of symptom management. In: Carroll-Johnson R (ed.), Oncology Nursing Forum. Pittsburgh: Oncology Nursing Press Inc.

Holmes S (1990a) Factors affecting the use of chemotherapeutic drugs. In: Cancer Chemotherapy. London: Austin Cornish Publishers Ltd.

Holmes S (1990b) The patient as an individual and use of chemotherapy in cancer treatment. In: Cancer Chemotherapy. London: Austin Cornish Publishers Ltd.

Holmes B (1996) Anxiety. In: Groenwald S, Goodman M, Yarbo C (eds), Cancer Symptom Management. Sudbury: Jones & Bartlett.

Howser D (1996) Alopecia. In: Groenwald S, Goodman M, Yarbo C (eds), Cancer Symptom Management. Sudbury: Jones & Bartlett.

Ingwersen K (1996) Cell cycle kinetics and antineoplastic agents. In: Burke MB, Wilkes GM, Ingwersen K, Bean C, Berg D (eds), Cancer Chemotherapy: A nursing process approach, 2nd edn. Boston, MA: Jones & Bartlett.

Jakubowski A (1996) Myelosuppression. In: Kirkwood J, Lotze M, Yasko J (eds), Current Cancer Therapeutics, 2nd edn. Philadelphia, PA: Churchill Livingstone.

Jenkins J (1996) Oncology nursing practice – the role of the nurse in support of progress in cancer treatment. In: Burke MB, Wilkes GM, Ingwersen K, Bean C, Berg D (eds), Cancer Chemotherapy: A nursing process approach, 2nd edn. Boston, MA: Jones & Bartlett.

Johnson M, Moroney C, Gay C (1997) Relieving nausea and vomiting in patients with cancer: a treatment algorithm. In: Carroll-Johnson R (ed.), Oncology Nursing Forum. Pittsburgh: Oncology Nursing Press, pp. 51–57 .

Klemn P, Hubbard S (1992) Infection. In: Groenwald S, Frogge M, Goodman M, Yarbo C (eds), Manifestations of Cancer and Cancer Treatment, 2nd edn. Boston, MA: Jones & Bartlett .

Kodish E, Singer P, Siegler M (1997) Ethical issues. In: DeVita V, Hellman S, Rosenberg S (eds), Cancer Principles and Practice of Oncology, 5th edn. Philadelphia, PA: Lippincott–Raven.

Kohne C (1999) 5-FU: Development of infusional 5-fluorouracil in the treatment of patients with metastatic colorectal cancer. (presentation summary). First European Conference: Perspectives in Colorectal Cancer. Bristol-Myers Squibb, 4–5 June: 33 .

Krook J, Moertel C, Grunderson L et al. (1991) Effective surgical adjuvant therapy for high risk rectal carcinoma. New England Journal of Medicine 324: 709–715.

Labianca R (1999) Adjuvant therapy for rectal cancer: the role of chemotherapy. In: Progress in Colorectal Cancer. London: Mediscript.

Lembersky B, Posner M (1996) Gastrointestinal toxicities. In: Kirkwood J, Lotze M, Yasko J (eds), Current Cancer Therapeutics, 2nd edn. Philadelphia, PA: Churchill Livingstone.

Leydon G, Boulton M, Moynihan C et al. (2000) Cancer patients' information needs and information seeking behaviour: in depth interview study. British Medical Journal 320: 909–913.

Linn E (1998) Diarrhoea. In: Yasko J (ed.), Nursing Management of Symptoms Associated with Chemotherapy, 4th edn. Bala Cynwyd, PA: Meniscus Health Care Communications.

Loprinzi C, Ghosh C, Camoriano J (1997) Phase II controlled evaluation of sucralfate to alleviate stomatitis in patients receiving fluorouracil based chemotherapy. Journal of Clinical Oncology 15: 1235–1238.

Lowry M (1995) Evaluating a patient teaching programme. Professional Nurse 11: 116–119.

Mahood D, Dose A, Loprinzi C (1991) Inhibition of fluorouracil induced stomatitis oral cryotherapy. Journal of Clinical Oncology 9: 449–452.

Mallett J, Bailey C (1996) Cytotoxic drugs: handling and administration In: The Royal Marsden NHS Trust Manual of Clinical Nursing Procedures. 4th edn. Oxford: Blackwell Science.

Mallett J, Dougherty L (2000) Vascular access therapy. In: The Royal Marsden Manual of Clinical Procedures. 5th edn. Oxford: Blackwell Science.

Meluch A, Hainsworth J, Thomas M et al. (1997) Preoperative therapy with paclitaxel, carboplatin, 5-FU and radiation yields 69% pathologic complete response (CR) rate in the treatment of local esophageal carcinoma. American Society of Clinical Oncology 16: 927.

Meropol N, Creaven J, Petrelli N (1995) Metastatic colorectal cancer: advances in biochemical modulation and new drug development. Seminars in Oncology 22: 509–524.

Miller S (1998) Stomatitis and oesophagitis. In: Yasko J (ed.), Nursing Management of Symptoms Associated with Chemotherapy 4th edn. Bala Cynwyd, PA: Meniscus Health Care Communications.

Minna J, Higgins G, Glatstein E (1984) Cancer of the lung. In: DeVita V, Hellman S, Rosenberg S (eds), Cancer Principles and Practice of Oncology, 5th edn. Philadelphia, PA: Lippincott–Raven.

Neoptolemos JP, Stocken DD, Dunn JA, Buckles J, Deakin M, Sutton R, Imrie C, Kerr DJ, Buchler for the members of ESPAC. Influence of the type of surgery and surgical complications in the ESPAC-1 adjuvant trial. British Journal of Surgery 89: 35 (abstract).

Nicolson M, Webb A, Cunningham D et al. (1995) Cisplatin and protracted venous infusion of 5-fluorouracil (cf) – good symptom relief with low toxicity in advanced pancreatic carcinoma. Annals of Oncology 6: 801–804.

Nightingale C, Norman A, Cunningham D, Young J, Webb A, Filshie J (1996) A prospective analysis of 949 long-term central venous access catheters for ambulatory chemotherapy in patients with gastrointestinal malignancy. European Journal of Cancer 33: 398–403.

O'Connell M, Mailliard J, Kahn M et al. (1997) Controlled trial of fluorouracil and low-dose leucovorin given for 6 months as post-operative adjuvant therapy for colon cancer. Journal of Clinical Oncology 15: 246–250.

Payne D, Massie M (1998) Depression and anxiety. In: Berger A, Portenoy R, Weissman D (eds), Principles and Practice of Supportive Oncology. Philadelphia, PA: Lippincott-Raven.

Pisters K, Kris M (1998) Treatment related to nausea and vomiting. In: Berger A, Portenoy R, Weissman D (eds), Principles and Practice of Supportive Oncology. Philadelphia: Lippincott-Raven.

Portenoy R, Miaskowski C (1998) Assessment and management of cancer related fatigue. In: Berger A, Portenoy R, Weissman D (eds), Principles and Practice of Supportive Oncology. Philadelphia: Lippincott-Raven.

Reville B, Almadrones L (1989) Continuous infusion chemotherapy in the ambulatory setting: The nurse's role in patient selection and education. Oncology Nursing Forum 16: 529-535.

Russell RCG, Ross P, Cunningham D (2002) Cancer of the Pancreas. In: Souhami RL, Tannok P, Hohenberger P, Horiot J-C (eds) The Oxford Book of Oncology, 2nd edn. Oxford: Oxford University Press.

Ross P, Norman A, Cunningham D et al. (1997) A prospective randomised trial of protracted venous infusion (PVI) 5-FU with or without mitomycin C (MMC) in advanced colorectal cancer. Annals of Oncology 8: 95-1001.

Ross P, Rao S, Cunningham D (1998) Chemotherapy of Oesphago-Gastric Cancer. Pathology Oncology Research. Philadelphia, PA: Saunders & Co. Ltd.

Roth J, Putnam J, Rich T, Forastiere A (1997) Cancers of the gastrointestinal tract – cancer of the esophagus. In: DeVita V, Hellman S, Rosenberg S (eds), Cancer Principles and Practice of Oncology, 5th edn. Philadelphia, PA: Lippincott-Raven.

Schafer S (1998) Infection due to leukopenia In: Yasko J (ed.), Nursing Management of Symptoms Associated with Chemotherapy, 4th edn. Bala Cynwyd, PA: Meniscus Health Care Communications.

Scheithauer W, Rosen H, Kornek G-V, Sebesta C, Depisch D (1993) Randomised comparison of combination chemotherapy plus supportive care with supportive care alone in patients with metastatic colorectal cancer. British Medical Journal 306: 752-755.

Schulmeister L (1992) An overview of continuous infusion chemotherapy. Journal of Intravenous Nursing 15: 315-321.

Seipp C (1998) Hair loss. In: DeVita V, Hellman S, Rosenberg S (eds), Cancer Principles and Practice of Oncology, 5th edn. Philadelphia, PA: Lippincott-Raven.

Shapiro R (1998) Informed consent. In: Berger A, Portenoy R, Weissman D (eds), Principles and Practice of Supportive Oncology. Philadelphia, PA: Lippincott-Raven.

Simon R (1997) Clinical trials in cancer – design and analysis of clinical trials In: DeVita V, Hellman S, Rosenberg S (eds), Cancer Principles and Practice of Oncology, 5th edn. Philadelphia, PA: Lippincott-Raven.

Sumpter K, Cunningham D (1998) Adjuvant chemotherapy in colorectal cancer (editorial). In: Progress in Colorectal Cancer. London: Mediscript.

Tanghe A, Evers G, Paridaens R (1998) Nurses' assessments of symptom occurrence and symptom distress in chemotherapy patients. European Journal of Oncology Nursing 2: 14-16.

Taplin S, Blanke C, Baughman C (1997) Nursing care strategies for the management of side effects in patients treated for colorectal cancer. Seminars in Oncology 24(5 suppl 18): S18-64-S18-70.

Taylor I, Goldberg, Garcia-Aguilar (1999) Treatment of the primary disease – colorectal cancer. In: Fast Facts. Indispensable guides to clinical practice. Oxford: Health Press.

Tempero M, Rasmussen B (1996) Upper gastrointestinal cancer. In: Kirkwood J, Lotze M, Yasko J (eds), Current Cancer Therapeutics, 2nd edn. Philadelphia, PA: Churchill Livingstone.

Van Cutsem E, Cunningham D, Hoff PM, Maroun J (2001) Thymidine Phosphorylase (TP) Activation: Convenience Through Innovation. The Oncologist Vol. 6 (supplement 4): 3–11.

Webb A, Cunningham D, Scargffe JH, Harper P, Norman A, Joffe JK (1997) Prospective randomised trial comparing epirubicin, cisplatin and flourouracil versus flourouracil, doxorubicin and methotrexate in advanced oesophagogastric cancer. Journal of Clinical Oncology 15(1): 261–267.

Whitman-Obert H (1996) Patient information handouts: taking care of yourself – a self help guide for patients with cancer. Oncology Nursing Forum 23: 1443–1445.

Winningham M (1996) Fatigue. In: Groenwald S, Goodman M, Yarbo C (eds), Cancer Symptom Management. Sudbury: Jones & Bartlett.

Wilkes G (1996) Potential toxicities and nursing management. In: Burke MB, Wilkes GM, Ingwersen K, Bean C, Berg D (eds), Cancer Chemotherapy: A nursing process approach, 2nd edn. Boston, MA: Jones & Bartlett.

World Health Organization (1997) WHO Handbook for Cancer Treatment. WHO Offset Publication, No. 48. Geneva: WHO.

Yarden Y, Ullrich A (1988) Growth factor receptor Tyrosine Kinases. Annual Review Biochemistry 57: 378–443.

CHAPTER 10

Symptom management and palliative care

JULIE MACDONALD AND TRACEY MCCREADY

One of the greatest challenges in cancer and palliative care for patients, their families and healthcare workers is to recognize and adapt to the changing nature of the disease as its impetus changes from curative treatment to restorative treatment and from care to palliative care. Schon, in 1993, when discussing the sociology of death, comments that there is no tangible boundary between the end of mainstream treatment and the beginning of dying. Schon goes on to say that dying will begin in the larger context of an already existing illness for which curative treatment is ongoing. Thus, although the introduction of palliative care might pose a challenge to health professionals, given that disease eradication is still in many cases the goal, the palliative care approach must be introduced from the time of diagnosis and not just when transitions in treatment occur.

The purpose of this chapter is to give the health professional an overview of pain and fatigue in cancer (other symptoms are discussed in other chapters), presenting the rationale for interventions, emphasizing the nursing role and offering practical applications. The importance of working in partnership with patients and their families in order to offer excellent care along the disease continuum is also discussed.

The philosophy of palliative care

Palliative care is 'the active, total care of patients whose disease no longer responds to curative treatment and for whom the goal must be the best quality of life for them and their families (World Health Organization, 1994). The Calman–Hine recommendations (Department of Health, 1995) acknowledge the centrality of palliative care in relation to cancer patients, suggesting that palliative care should be incorporated in a seamless way into the care of cancer patients from the time of diagnosis.

Palliative care provision can broadly be divided into two categories: non-specialist and specialist. Non-specialist palliative care should in theory be provided by all disciplines who are advised and given practical support by specialists in palliative care although specialist palliative care is usually practised by someone who has acquired specific qualifications in the area or has considerable experience in caring for dying people and their families.

It is important to remember that palliative care is not about hospices – it is a philosophy of care that can be delivered in any setting. It aims to relieve unpleasant symptoms and improve the quality of life for all those with non-curable conditions.

Aims of palliative care

Palliative care should not be seen as crisis intervention and should be applied long before this arises. Palliative care should enable dying people to be pain free and experience a dignified death. Its aims are:

- To provide symptom control and pain relief.
- To create a support system for dying people, addressing the social, emotional, spiritual and practical needs in an individualized way, while allowing them choice.
- To provide emotional, spiritual and practical care for the dying person's family and friends from the time of diagnosis until after death.
- To establish a team with good communication between them, including the dying person and his or her family.
- To provide support and advice for those caring for dying people.

Communication in palliative care

The literature over the past 10 years clearly highlights that the common practices surrounding death at the beginning of the twentieth century, such as caring for the dying person at home, burial rituals and mourning, are given little recognition as we enter the twenty-first century (Copp, 1994). It is therefore not surprising that knowing what to do and what to say when confronted by a palliative care patient and their family is challenging to many nurses and other healthcare professionals (Cooley, 2000). The fear of the reactions of the patient or family is often a concern for the health professional within palliative care and in any situation where one has to break bad news.

Research evidence makes strong links between quality of communication by healthcare providers and quality of life for cancer patients throughout the cancer journey. Much research has as its focus the medical encounter, and findings suggest that a constructive relationship between physician and patient is consistent with better coping and satisfaction with treatment protocols, improved information exchange, increased accrual into clinical trials, and improved rapport and patient understanding (Ruckdeschel et al., 1996). Therefore, it is clear that communication can have a direct effect on quality of life for the cancer patient. Furthermore, constructive and positive communications in cancer care have been linked with a sense of control, active information-seeking behaviours, disclosing feelings and a search for meaning (Northouse and Northouse, 1987).

Interventions for communication

In 1991 Simpson et al. presented explanations of how quality of healthcare communication can be linked to specific illness-related outcomes. Explanation and understanding of patient concerns, even if they cannot be resolved, result in significant anxiety reduction. Similarly, greater participation in care results in better compliance and better information results in decreased psychological distress. Reduction in anxiety and distress has a direct effect on pain and symptom control.

Patients and their families can feel powerless within the cancer care system; they feel vulnerable to the healthcare professionals who have control over how decisions and resources in the system are determined (Thorne, 1985). Good communication helps patients and their families to be empowered and to cope with their illness in partnership with healthcare professionals. Partnership in care fosters trust and reduces vulnerability and anxiety.

According to Cooley (2000), understanding that the patient's emotional state is individual rather than a stage in a process may enable more effective nurse–patient interaction. She goes on to say that the interaction between the patient and family and the professional carer can influence the feelings of satisfaction at the standard of care being delivered. Poor communication between professionals and between the nurse and his or her patient can lead to feelings of frustration and irritation, causing anxiety and stress. It is up to healthcare professionals to empower their patients and families on the cancer journey, to have enough information and to foster a trusting relationship that enables the two to walk the cancer pathway together.

Psychosocial aspects of palliative care

In the last quarter of the twentieth century, research developments into the subjective nature of cancer, quality-of-life issues and delivery of care show that the social domain in which cancer is lived can affect the way people cope with cancer and the meaning it has in their lives. This social arena operates on different levels: in healthcare encounters, family life, encounters in the social world and the public media, and the ideological structures underlying the way healthcare services are delivered (Thorne, 1999).

People with cancer often experience psychosocial problems relating to the diagnosis, treatment and prognosis of the disease (Bottomley, 1997b). According to Barraclough (1997) 10–20% of patients go on to develop formal psychiatric disorders, making the cancer journey even more difficult both for themselves and for their families. Patients are faced with a life-threatening condition, associated with fear of the unknown, unpleasant treatment, side effects and loss of self-esteem (Cook, 1999). Cancer disrupts feelings, attitudes and relationships, and is seen as a metaphor for death (Corner, 1993).

Klemm et al. (2000) conducted a study to describe the most common and most intense demands of the illness in people with colorectal cancer. The results of the study showed that demands of illness were greatest in the personal meaning domain – 93% of participants reported that they thought about the value of life and how long they might live. The 10 most intense demands were predominately psychosocial and existential concerns.

Self-concept becomes challenged by the dependency of the patient on others, loss of social interaction, and the patients' decreasing ability to help themselves and others (Courtans et al.,

1996). The diagnosis, treatment and prognosis of cancer deny the security and certainty of patients' lives and can take away their control over their own destiny. People with a cancer can struggle to come to terms with the diagnosis, which can lead to anger and negative thinking. Generalized feelings of depression can ensue, causing the individual to become withdrawn, especially if feelings are not expressed openly and dealt with effectively (Saunders, 1995). Even if those feelings are externalized, if they are dealt with ineffectively this can lead to isolation, while those close to the patient fail to understand what is happening.

Patients with cancer may start reviewing their lives and, rather than looking at achievements, they may find that they are concentrating on their failings and unfulfilled ambitions. As the patient nears death, he or she may also be faced with the worry of those being left behind. In 'Man's search for meaning', Frankl (1963) drew attention to the search for meaning in one's life. He believed that meaning is a basic human need necessary for human fulfilment, but that the journey is often postponed until one faces mortality, experiences suffering or undergoes a life-changing experience (Ferrell et al., 1999).

Ferrell et al. (1995) identified a process of making meaning out of the cancer experience:

- Identifying a causal attribution – to prevent saying 'why me?'. The cancer may be familial, the patient may have smoked – any reason.
- Finding benefits of the disease and suffering – looking for the positive, families brought together.
- Making downward social comparisons – there are always people worse off than ourselves.
- Placing the cancer experience within the larger context of life – reprioritizing future life goals and reflecting on previous achievements.

The outcomes associated with making meaning of the cancer experience include:

- Positive coping – being empowered and in control.
- Increased hopefulness – for a future living and coping with cancer.
- Transcendence – one can look positively at life and achievements and be fulfilled.

Untreated symptoms such as uncontrolled pain and over-whelming suffering can hinder the ability to make sense of or give meaning to the illness. Thus, one goal of nursing is to enhance the patient's and family's ability to make meaning out of cancer (Ferrell et al., 1999).

Interventions for psychosocial care

Jenkinson (1996) talks about the nurse as being a 'significant other' to his or her patients. A significant other is someone to whom we refer – whose comments, opinions and reactions are of particular significance to us. Friends, partners, family members, parents and teachers are often recognized as being significant, because it is the views and behaviours of these people that are particularly valued and therefore tend to have the greatest impact. Many nurses fail to realize their potential to be a significant other or feel unable to meet the demands of the role, because of either a perceived lack of ability or simply a lack of time. As a result, there is a danger that nurses working in busy wards may prefer to relinquish the responsibility of psychological care to specialist nurses, who will see the patient only periodically.

Cooley (2000, pp. 602–3) says about the assessment of palliative care patients:

> without appropriate communication skills, eliciting a useful assessment becomes difficult. The assessment tends to be based on the physical care needs of the patient and does not encompass the psychological, social, sexual or cultural issues that make up the whole patient.

In addition to asking routine questions about physical symptoms, nurses should get into the habit of asking general therapeutic questions aimed at assessing spiritual and psychosocial issues (Klemm et al., 2000).

Maleham (1999) found that staff perceived themselves as just getting by with the psychological aspects of care and did not always know where to refer patients with psychological difficulties. However, quite often nurses are the only individuals present when patients feel the need for support. This places them in a position where it is necessary for them to be able to offer this support at a time when it is most needed. (Cook, 1999)

If one addresses the perceived inadequacies of the nurse with regard to psychosocial support for the cancer patient, support for the nurse needs to be addressed to enable him or her adequately to assess and care holistically for the cancer patient.

This support can take several forms:

- Education on psychosocial issues
- Multidisciplinary staff support
- Liaison with specialist nurses
- Clinical supervision.

Bottorff et al. (1995), in their work exploring the work of cancer nurses, observed various combinations of comforting strategies. The strategies include:

- Helping patients put experiences into perspective – providing information and using gentle humour.
- Helping them to stay in control – empowering the patient with information and offering a choice where possible.
- Providing opportunities for them to function as normally as possible – maximizing or restoring body function.
- Providing emotional support – with excellent interpersonal skills, truly empathizing with the patient.

This work sums up quite nicely the expectation that we would have of any nurse caring for a cancer patient, given the right amount of support.

> Therapeutic cancer nursing should be offered within the context of care that is participative, collaborative and empowering of people with cancer, their families and carers.
>
> Corner (1993)

Pain and symptom management

Of the many symptoms of cancer, pain is often the most feared, as a result of the fact that unrelieved pain affects every aspect of a person's life. Studies indicate that cancer pain is synonymous with anxiety, fatigue, emotional distress, mood disorders, depression, fewer social interactions and altered family activities (Dorepaal et al., 1989). Relief of pain is essential to improve the quality of life for patients with cancer, yet cancer-related pain is often poorly treated resulting in unnecessary suffering.

The literature suggests that nurses often do not possess sufficient knowledge with which to nurse patients in pain and that pain control remains inadequate (Clarke et al., 1996; McCaffery and

Ferrell, 1997; Drayer et al., 1999). The World Health Organization states that pain can be controlled in 70-90% of cancer patients using relatively inexpensive and simple methods (WHO, 1996); however, it has been estimated that adequate control of pain is achieved in only 50% of patients in Western societies (Hanks, 1994). This section aims to give the reader an overview of pain, including assessment and principles of management. The reader is guided to the numerous books available for in-depth knowledge of physiology and pharmacology.

Acute pain

Acute pain has a definite onset, usually as a result of an injury or illness, and its duration is limited and predictable. It is often accompanied by signs of anxiety and clinical signs of tachycardia, tachypnoea, sweating, dilated pupils and pallor. These signs are considered characteristic of individuals in pain (Figure 10.1).

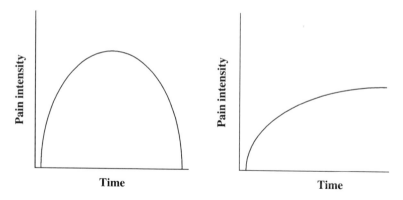

Figure 10.1 Variation between acute and chronic pain over time. (From Woodruff, 1996.)

Chronic pain

Chronic pain differs from acute pain in that it results from a chronic pathological process. The onset is gradual over time and it can become progressively more severe. Individuals often appear depressed or withdrawn and are frequently described as not looking like 'someone in pain'.

Nurses will care for patients experiencing different types of pain; the most common types are defined as follows.

Neuropathic pain

This pain, also called neurogenic or deafferentation pain, is often hard for patients and staff to understand because there is no obvious noxious stimulus present. This type of pain is the result of current or past damage to the peripheral and/or central nervous system. It can be very unpleasant and long lasting, resulting in loss of sleep, and is described in various ways. Patients often say it is burning, aching or dull in type; however, sharp shooting pains can also be experienced plus numbness. Some patients cannot bear clothing to touch the affected area.

Somatic pain

Somatic pain refers to pain in the musculoskeletal system, namely, bones, periosteum, tendons and fascia.

Visceral pain

This is pain in the internal organs. Twisting and distension affect internal organs such as the gut and this causes the pain. Acute visceral pain is often very intense, dull and aching; it is vaguely localized and accompanied by rigid abdominal muscles (guarding), pallor and sweating. Small amounts of visceral pain lead to dramatic autonomic activity (Cervero, 1991). The pain a person experiences is disproportionate to the internal damage. An important point to note is that visceral pain leads to referred pain.

Pain and advanced cancer are not synonymous. Although three-quarters of patients experience pain, a quarter do not (Twycross, 1997). Multiple concurrent pains are common in those who have pain (Figure 10.2):

- One-third will have a single pain
- One-third will have two pains
- One-third will have three or more pains.

Not all cancer pain is the result of the actual cancer. According to Woodruff (1996):

- 70% is caused by tumour involvement
- 20% is associated with treatment
- <10% is the result of general illness but not cancer
- <10% is unrelated to the cancer or its treatment.

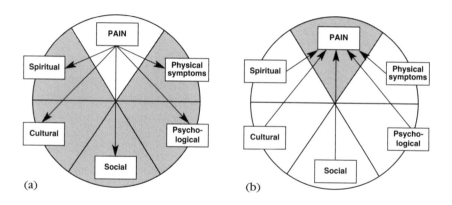

Figure 10.2 Interdependence of the various causes of suffering: (a) unrelieved pain may cause or aggravate problems related to any of the other aspects of suffering; (b) unresolved or untreated problems related to any of the other causes of suffering may cause or aggravate pain. (From Woodruff, 1996.)

Total pain

When discussing pain, it is important to be aware that we should not just be looking at it as a physical dimension. Saunders (1967) introduced the concept of total pain to highlight that pain is multidimensional, and that non-physical as well as physical aspects must be addressed.

Pain is also associated with suffering. Unrelieved pain may exacerbate other physical symptoms and vice versa. Problems in other areas can also aggravate pain. These problems need addressing if pain is to be effectively managed, and looking at the individuals and their families and caring for them in a holistic way can do this best (Figure 10.3).

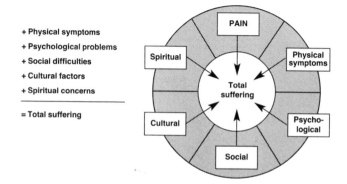

Figure 10.3 Attributes from the whole person are associated with total suffering.

Perception of pain

Pain is 'whatever the experiencing person says it is, existing whenever the experiencing person says it does' (McCaffery and Beebe, 1989). Pain is always subjective. It is important to be aware that other physical symptoms will aggravate the perception of pain, so palliation of other symptoms is essential to improve pain control. Other factors can also affect pain; looking at the individual holistically will ensure that none of these issues is missed.

Psychological problems

These are the most common factors aggravating perception of pain and a failure to recognize and treat psychological distress will worsen an individual's pain. Some clinical features of psychological distress are anxiety, depression and despair. The management of these problems is aimed at helping patients to develop their adaptive and coping mechanisms (Woodruff, 1996) and this needs to be individualized for each patient. Counselling could be valuable. Support groups provide both emotional and social support; they may help pain control and reduce anxiety and depression (Bottomley, 1997a).

Social difficulties

Individuals with cancer are usually members of families and have other social networks. This means that they have social and financial responsibilities. Problems in any of these areas, e.g. financial hardship or relationship problems, can lead to isolation and/or withdrawal, and may mean that pain is harder to control.

Cultural factors

It is important to be aware that different cultures have varying degrees of acceptance of pain – ranging from stoicism to severe anxiety and depression, with some writers suggesting that people in Western cultures have a lower tolerance of pain (Illich, 1976; Menges, 1984). Attitudes to pain relief and palliative care also vary. Communication can be made difficult because of language barriers. Culturally sensitive management is essential and can best be achieved by being knowledgeable about the culture and an individual's perception of pain. Interpreters can be used to help with communication.

Spiritual factors

This must not be confused with religion; every individual has his or her own spirituality which centres on meaning and existence. An individual may have regrets or guilt about past events, e.g. about relationships or missed opportunities, and they may feel that now there is no time to rectify these. Allowing them time to talk or tell their story can help and go some way to relieving their distress. For those who observe religious practices, there may be specific problems, e.g. they may believe that their disease is a punishment. Highfield (1992) highlighted that nurses do not assess patients' spiritual needs, but nurses must ensure that this aspect is not overlooked, by discussing it when planning a programme of care and not being afraid to enlist the help of others, e.g. ministers of religion (Hawthorn and Redmond, 1998)

Assessment of pain

Successful management of pain depends on an accurate systemic assessment (de Wit et al., 1999). Recent reviews have, however, found little evidence that this takes place and that assessment is problematic and inconsistent (McCaffery and Ferrell, 1997; de Rond et al., 1999). Assessment needs to be comprehensive and to include all aspects of pain, not just the severity. An accurate assessment of pain relies on nurses believing the patients' pain rating. Implementation of therapeutic control is not always appropriate to the pain rating, suggesting that nurses may not accept patients' reporting of their own pain (McCaffery and Ferrell, 1997).

Barriers to adequate assessment

Incorrect interpretation of non-verbal cues can contribute to poor assessment. Nurses may assume that, if patients look comfortable or are sleeping, they must be pain free because individuals in pain are expected to exhibit certain behaviours and physiological signs. Some pain control behaviours such as watching television, chatting or participating in activities can also be interpreted as signs that the patient is not in pain (Redd et al., 2001).

Those who experience more expressible pain behaviours such as crying, moaning or facial expressions of suffering can be perceived by nurses as being more distressed than the stoic patient (Von Baeyer et al., 1984). Assessment of pain is further complicated by nurses assuming that patients will complain of pain, whereas patients expect the nurse to enquire about their pain (Seers, 1987; Franke and Theeuwen, 1994). Poor communication on the part of the nurse and patients can hinder assessment. Difficulties can arise when patients are unable to find the words to describe the pain adequately.

Wilkinson (1991) studied nurses communicating with cancer patients and found that they carried out very superficial assessments; thus interventions were planned on the basis of incomplete information. Just as the patient's culture affects the perception of pain, the nurse's own cultural background may also influence the degree to which she or he infers suffering in patients. There is evidence that nurses from various backgrounds differ in their inferences of both physical pain and psychological distress (Davitz and Davitz, 1985; McCaffery and Ferrell, 1997).

Assessment tools

A comprehensive assessment tool is essential. There are many different kinds of instruments for assessing the intensity and type of pain, and nurses are more knowledgeable than physicians or pharmacists in pain assessment (Furstenburg et al., 1998). The process of assessment should include facilitating the patients to tell their own story through their own perspective (Webb, 1992). The simplest measures of pain, and those most widely used, are the visual analogue scale (VAS) and the verbal pain rating scale. The VAS is an easy and simple tool for the assessment of pain and the measurement of pain intensity. It is important that the same kind of instrument is always used with the same patient. Daily pain ratings are essential to ensure continuity and it is important that the information is documented. Evidence shows that recording of ratings is inconsistent (Graffam, 1990) (Figure 10.4).

Either patients or nurse can complete pictorial records of the site of pain (Figure 10.5). However, it should be noted that patients and nurses differ in their assessment of the most intense level of pain suffered by patients, with nurses believing that their patients accept and tolerate more pain than the patients themselves say is the case (Hovi and Lauri, 1999).

Despite the benefits of assessing pain, many nurses resist using the tools. Common criticisms are that using them takes

Visual analogue scale

Instruction: mark on the line below how strong your pain is

No pain ———————————————— Worst possible pain

Numerical rating scale

Instruction: on a scale of 1 to 10, how strong is your pain?

No pain = 0 – 1 – 2 – 3 – 4 – 5 – 6 – 7 – 8 – 9 – 10 = Worst pain possible

Verbal descriptor scale

Instruction: which word best describes your pain?

None   Mild   Moderate   Severe   Excruciating

Figure 10.4 Self-report measures for pain severity. (From Woodruff, 1996.)

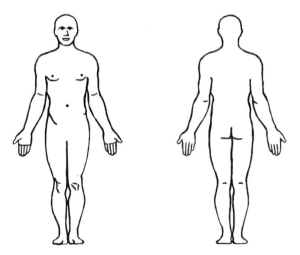

Figure 10.5 Pictorial pain record: the patient is asked to indicate the site of the pain or it may be completed by the examining doctor or nurse. (From Woodruff, 1996.)

too long and some nurses feel that their own judgement is satisfactory. However, nursing a patient with unmanaged pain takes
far longer, so time taken to assess it is worth while. Relying on
one's own judgement can be dangerous if the practitioner is a
novice in this field because information may be missed; use of a
tool can help ensure that nothing is missed (Gordon, 1987). It is
also important to use a tool to ensure consistency, because the
same nurse is not on duty 24 hours a day 7 days a week. Others
argue that assessment tools in use are not relevant to their clinical area, in which case the tools can be adapted to suit it.

Just carrying out an assessment is pointless unless the information obtained is used in clinical decision-making. Just as a
finding that a patient has high blood pressure or temperature
will trigger the nurse to take action, so too should a high pain
assessment score. Tools are also helpful in evaluating the effectiveness of the pain management programme.

Management of pain

Good communication with both the patient and other members
of the caring team will ensure a coordinated approach to pain
control. It is essential to reassure the patient that the pain can be
relieved. Patients are entitled to expect effective pain management and a total absence of pain wherever possible. As all
aspects of pain need to be addressed, a multidisciplinary
approach should be employed.

As pain becomes worse, and it occupies a person's whole
attention, other interventions can be used. Evidence shows that
non-pharmacological interventions are effective in the management of pain and nurses should consider using these in pain
management (Sindhu, 1996; Wallace, 1997); despite this, nurses
tend not to use these approaches (Ferrell et al., 1991a; Franke et
al., 1996). Diversional activities can be used because they do
more than just pass the time – nurses can encourage patients to
watch television, read or converse. If pain persists, it may be
necessary to modify a patient's way of life and environment. The
help of the physiotherapist and occupational therapist is often
valuable.

The multifaceted nature of pain means that it is unlikely that
pharmacological interventions will give total relief. Nurses can
use other pain control interventions, such as distraction,
massage or the application of heat, in their everyday practice to

benefit patients. Poor positioning can also exacerbate pain; important interventions include helping a patient who is bed bound to maintain a comfortable position with the use of pillows and other supports, and minimizing the number of times that they have to move (Hawthorn and Redmond, 1998). Evidence shows, however, that nurses tend not to do this (Ferrell et al., 1991a; Fothergill-Bourbonnais and Wilson Barnett, 1992; Franke et al., 1996).

Non-pharmacological interventions for pain managment

Massage

Massage has been used as a therapeutic intervention for thousands of years. It can have a direct physiological effect on pain, reducing muscle spasm and tension. Carers can be taught simple massage techniques, which can help overcome feelings of helplessness. Before attempting to use massage, it must first be ascertained whether touch is acceptable to the patient because it may cause anxiety and discomfort in those who dislike physical touch (Hawthorn and Redmond, 1998). Concern has been expressed that massage may encourage the spread of cancer (McNamara, 1994); however, although there is no evidence to support this belief, it is not wise to massage directly over a palpable tumour or an area undergoing radiotherapy.

Reflexology

Reflexology is a treatment that has its roots in massage. It can be performed on the feet or hands and used to treat various disorders. Application of gentle pressure to these areas may reduce pain and anxiety. Basic foot massage can be taught to carers and this allows them to be involved in care (Whitlock, 1999).

Heat treatment

Heat treatment can be used effectively to relieve pain, offering a simple and cost-effective non-pharmacological intervention for pain (Hawthorn and Redmond, 1998). The superficial application of heat increases the blood flow to skin and superficial organs, which will improve tissue oxygenation and nutrition and aid the elimination of pain-causing substances (Hawthorn and Redmond, 1998, p. 213). It is of particular benefit in the treatment of muscle spasms and musculoskeletal discomforts, which are associated with immobility and debility. As heat treatment can cause tissue damage, care should be taken where there is diminished sensation or paralysis; it should also be avoided in the presence of infection. Heat treatment can be achieved with hot packs, hot water bottles, electric heating pads, radiant heat lamps and hydrotherapy.

Although there is still controversy about the use of superficial heat in cancer patients, with some expressing concern that it facilitates tumour growth and metastatic spread, evidence to support this view is limited and the use of superficial heat to control pain can still be recommended (Jacox et al., 1994).

Cold therapy

Cold therapy, the superficial application of cold, causes vaso-constriction of the skin blood vessels and helps prevent or reduce swelling after injury. It can also decrease the production of pain-causing metabolites and conduction in pain fibres (Ernst and Fialka, 1994). Cold is thought to be more effective, have a shorter duration of application, work more quickly and produce a longer-lasting effect than heat (Hawthorn and Redmond, 1998). Unfortunately, many people are averse to cold and find heat much more acceptable (McCaffery, 1990). Cold therapy can be applied in the form of icepacks, ethyl chloride spray or immersion in iced water. The application of both extreme heat and cold is contraindicated in areas that have previously been treated with radiotherapy (Hawthorn and Redmond, 1998).

Music therapy

According to Larsen-Beck (1991), music can ameliorate pain by means of distraction, reduction of anxiety, counterstimulation and increased feelings of control. This finding supports earlier work, also on oncology patients by Zimmerman and colleagues (1989). Nurses can help by offering patients a range of different music to listen to, with headphones to block out distracting noise.

Environment

An unpleasant environment and loss of privacy have been cited as factors contributing to pain (Faggerhaugh and Strauss, 1977; Wainwright, 1985). Allowing patients control over lighting, temperature and ventilation can help, as can affording them privacy. It may be difficult for patients to express their pain in a busy ward and this makes assessment difficult. A pleasant environment facilitates rest and can help in the alleviation of pain (Fordham and Dunn, 1994). Achieving this in a hospital is difficult; however, this should not deter health professionals from trying.

Education of patients and families

The nurse has a pivotal role to play in the education of patients and families. Myths and misconceptions about pain and treatment abound and this can result in patients either refusing to take analgesics or increasing the dose. Patients who receive drug-related education have improved pain relief, better compliance with pain medication regimens and less concern about taking opiates than patients who have not received such education (Rimer et al., 1992). Families also have a need for information, especially if they are involved in the care of the patient at home. Family members often have to decide what pain medication to give, how much to give and when to give it (Ferrell et al., 1991b). It is important to remember that their response to expressions of pain can ameliorate or exacerbate it, so patient and family education is an on-going process, not a one-off event.

Nurses need to give patients taking a number of different medications the following information:

- Written instructions to take home.
- Warning about possible side effects, because experiencing these when medication is first started may lead to a discontinuation.
- Contact telephone numbers, which patients should be advised to call if they have any concerns.

Analgesic programmes should be kept as simple as possible and any fears about dependence and addiction need to be discussed. Patients are often anxious when prescribed morphine, thinking that they will soon die or that nothing will be left when the pain gets worse. They need reassurance that morphine can be used for months or years and is compatible with a normal lifestyle, and that the therapeutic range is such that the dosage can be increased if necessary.

Principles of pharmacological pain relief

The principles of pain relief are covered in this section; again the reader is guided to books on pharmacology for more detailed guidance, e.g. Twycross (1994).

Satisfactory pain relief can be achieved in 95% of patients with cancer. It is best to aim for the following:

- Pain relief at night
- Pain relief at rest during the day
- Pain relief on movement (recognizing that this is not always possible).

The oral route is the preferred route and analgesics should be given regularly and prophylactically, never 'as required'. The WHO's three-step analgesic ladder (WHO, 1994) should be used (Figure 10.6). Woodruff (1996) suggests the following examples of drugs to be used at each stage:

Step 1: aspirin or non-steroidal anti-inflammatory drugs
Step 2: codeine or oxycodeine
Step 3: morphine or methadone.

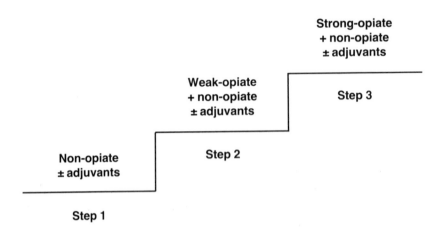

Figure 10.6 Analgesic ladder. (From WHO, 1994).

Adjuvant drugs

Adjuvant drugs should be used, e.g. laxatives are always required with morphine usage. An adjuvant drug is, strictly speaking, one that potentiates the action of another, e.g. an adjuvant anxiolytic may be given alongside an analgesic to reduce anxiety and this will also help pain relief.

Antidepressant drugs

Antidepressant drugs have also been shown to be analgesic for a wide variety of painful conditions, e.g. headache and chronic facial pain, and can be useful in patients with high levels of anxiety.

Steroids

Steroids reduce oedema and thus can be useful in relieving visceral pain and bone pain because they relieve pressure on compressed structures. The analgesic effect is accompanied by an increase in appetite and well-being.

Anticonvulsants

Anticonvulsants can be useful in the treatment of neuropathic pain, although the mechanism of action is unknown (Hawthorn and Redmond, 1998, pp. 176–183).

Although detailed description of all medication used to relieve pain is beyond the scope of this section, it is important that nurses have a good knowledge of pain medication. Hovi and Lauri (1999) found that nurses with poor knowledge of morphine and its use in pain management tended to underestimate the patients' most intense experiences of pain.

Points to be aware of are that morphine usage is dictated by therapeutic need, not by prognosis and, in cancer patients, it does not cause clinically important respiratory depression. The use of morphine does not, however, guarantee success in pain relief if the psychosocial aspects of care are ignored.

Cancer-related fatigue

Fatigue is a complex, multidimensional subjective experience and is today the most frequently reported symptom from patients with cancer (Magnusson et al., 1999). According to Porock (1999), the differences between 'normal fatigue' and cancer-related fatigue are most obvious when time is factored into the definition. Fatigue in palliative care patients is sustained and not relieved by rest. Porock (1999) goes on to describe fatigue as a symptom of disease expressed by the whole person, physically, mentally, emotionally and socially.

The subjective nature of fatigue brings with it descriptors such as: tiredness, weakness, exhaustion, lethargy, depression, malaise, etc., with patients often using metaphors to describe fatigue. In the study of Ferrell et al. (1996) on the experience of fatigue and its impact on quality of life, fatigue was described by one patient as feeling like 'wet cement'. One can only try to imagine the severity of the fatigue suffered in order to draw on such a metaphor. Ferrell's quotation from one of her patients used to name her study is 'bone tired', again an apt description of something that for most of us will resolve with a good night's sleep, but what of the cancer patient? 'Fatigue wastes time and time is precious' (Ferrell et al., 1996).

Cancer-related fatigue is chronic with a gradual, insidious onset, often with no identifiable cause and often bearing no relationship to activity levels. Acute fatigue, on the other hand, has a rapid onset, usually with an identifiable cause and is relieved by rest (Piper et al., 1987).

Fatigue is often assumed to accompany illness. When it prompts the patient to seek help, it is usually debilitating and affecting quality of life (Ferrell et al., 1996). Fatigue, along with weakness, has a tendency to increase as cancer progresses (Richardson and Ream, 1996). Effective treatment modalities for other symptoms such as nausea and vomiting and pain can induce and/or exacerbate fatigue.

Causes of cancer-related fatigue

Fatigue has many causes in both healthy individuals and those with a disease process such as cancer. It is unclear how pre-existing conditions, direct effects of cancer, symptoms related to cancer, effects of cancer treatment and the demands of dealing with cancer interact to produce or exacerbate fatigue (Winningham et al., 1994). The literature alludes to energy deficits measured against demands and how the cancer affects energy metabolism against energy expenditure (Richardson and Ream, 1999). Factors that predispose to or influence the severity of cancer-related fatigue can be categorized as disease related, personal and environmental (Porock, 1999).

Disease related

Research on the effects of different treatment modalities for cancer indicate that fatigue is a common side effect:

- Chemotherapy: 80–100% of patients (Richardson, 1995)
- Radiotherapy: up to 100% of patients (Fieler, 1997)
- Biotherapy: related to dose, being cumulative in nature (Brophy and Sharp, 1991)
- Surgery (Cimprich, 1992).

Evidence shows that treatments have a long-lasting effect on energy reserves and may be cumulative in nature (Porock, 1999). As well as metabolic changes, resulting from the disease process, requiring energy expenditure, the physical effort of undergoing diagnostic procedures and treatment can deplete energy reserves.

Personal and environmental factors

Ferrell et al. (1996) describe fatigue in relation to quality of life for patients with cancer and, along with Magnusson et al. (1999), discuss the multidimensional concept. Fatigue can impact on every part of the patient's life: physically affecting body function and physical well-being; psychologically linking with anxiety and depression (Ferrell et al., 1996); socially affecting the role of the patient within the family and the wider community; and spiritually heightening feelings of hopelessness and uncertainty.

The later work of Magnusson and colleagues (1999), a qualitative study to explore the experience of fatigue in cancer patients, describes fatigue as a process building on the holistic and subjective nature described in their previous work. They describe three major categories affecting fatigue:

1. Experience: of loss, need, psychological stress, emotional affect, abnormal weakness, difficulty in taking the initiative.
2. Consequences: social limitation, affected self-esteem, affected quality of life.
3. Actions: coping, adjusting activities to cope with symptoms and reprioritizing life goals.

When so much work has been done in other areas of symptom management, such as relief from nausea and pain control to improve quality of life in cancer and palliative care, what can be done to relieve fatigue and further improve quality of life for those with cancer and for those who care for them? Knowledge about the different expressions of fatigue is important in caring for patients with cancer (Magnusson et al., 1999). Lack of a formal definition for fatigue hinders the healthcare practitioner's understanding of it, which can result in poor communication; this creates difficulties in assessment and decision-making for interventions (Porock, 1999).

Assessment

Assessment of fatigue is often by way of a single item on a general assessment checklist. This results partly from its perceived seriousness as a true symptom of cancer by some healthcare professionals. There are, however, several fatigue inventories to aid assessment, as well as checklists and scales. The scale and inventory can be used in combination to assess and evaluate fatigue. The Rhoten fatigue scale gives a quick assessment that is easy to monitor; it is unidimensional and pragmatic, and permits comparisons over time (Rhoten, 1982, cited in Winningham, 1999). The Rhoten assessment tool consists of a 10-point scale similar to a pain assessment tool, where 0 = not tired/full of energy and 10 = total exhaustion; the patient is asked to use his or her own words to describe the points in between. It can be useful to take a fatigue inventory from the patient, to assess the impact of fatigue on activities of living and to open up conversation and give the patient time to reflect on levels of fatigue. A scale such as the Rhoten can very easily be incorporated into a general assessment procedure, and administered at the same time as a pain scale, e.g. giving it the high profile it deserves both with the healthcare professional and the patient.

Interventions for fatigue

Richardson and Ream (1999), in a review of the evidence available to guide the development of interventions to alleviate cancer-related fatigue, found that, without guidance, patients adopt common-sense strategies that generally prove unsuccessful in alleviating fatigue. Rest is the most frequently noted strategy, but this in itself can lead to the development of fatigue and weakness, and result in rapid and potentially irreversible losses in energy and function. Magnusson et al. (1999) refer to self-help activities, e.g. going to bed earlier, resting, exercising, planning daily activities, delegating household tasks and distractions. Richardson and Ream (1999) go on to discuss how theories that identify self-care actions that can reduce fatigue are becoming increasingly sophisticated. However, they point out the implications for nursing practice in that patients require guidance in managing cancer-related fatigue.

The literature on intervention strategies focuses on four main interventions: exercise, attention-restoring activities, preparatory education and psychosocial techniques.

Exercise

In studies on the benefits of a structured exercise programme, patients reported less fatigue and additional psychosocial benefits linked to a sense of well-being (Richardson and Ream, 1999). In a study on exercise in women with breast cancer, exercise decreased perceptions of fatigue and confirmed the benefits of aerobic activity (Winningham et al., 1985). Further research may be necessary before one could advocate a structured exercise programme in all cancer patients; however, encouraging more general exercise could meet the needs of the patient – encouraging some form of exercise two to three times daily, e.g. walking the dog, walking to the shop, swimming, gentle gardening, or even chair or bed exercises.

Attention-restoring activities

For attention-restoring activities, favourite activities and enjoyable pastimes are encouraged to prevent boredom and understimulation. Cimprich's work, in 1993, with a control group suggested that this intervention is effective and patients following a programme of activity had enhanced attentional capacity. It is important to remember that although patients have things/activities that they need to do, such as attending hospital and maintaining activities of daily living, they also have things that they want to do such as enjoyable pastimes. The family may need help in planning activities and rest periods in order to maintain a high quality of life.

Preparatory education

Preparatory education related to fatigue for cancer patients can alleviate the widely held perception that fatigue is an indication of disease progression, when that is not always the case, or that treatment may be ineffective (Richardson and Ream, 1999). Patients with fatigue can lose control of their everyday activities, partly as a result of anxiety. By empowering the patient and the family, giving them the information they need and educating them, they may have the power to regain control.

Psychosocial techniques

The literature advocates the benefits of psychosocial intervention to relieve fatigue in cancer sufferers. However, the blanket approach is not advocated; intervention should be tailored to the individual needs of the patient, with selective services targeted at those at risk of psychological morbidity. Services may include relaxation, guided imagery, music therapy and time management, to give a few examples.

The nurse can help the patient and the family build a framework for the management of fatigue. By empowering the patient with the knowledge available on cancer-related fatigue, activity and rest can be incorporated into activities of daily living. Psychosocial intervention at a basic level would follow by being involved with the patient's management. Intervention could be increased as necessary, depending on the patient's need. 'Cancer related fatigue is a whole body experience' (Porock, 1999). Management of fatigue needs to be holistic, working in partnership with the patient and his or her family, taking account of the disease trajectory, its symptoms and interventions, in order to promote the highest quality of life possible.

Conclusion

There is evidence to suggest that the quality of the cancer experience affects not only the patient, but also those close to them. A consistent concern of families is the need for the patient to receive pain relief and adequate comfort care (Ferrell et al., 1991b). Families who witness the suffering or uncontrolled pain of a relative experience suffering themselves (Kristjanson and Avery, 1994). The authors hope that this chapter has inspired the reader to work closely with colleagues, patients and their families to develop interpersonal skills and use evidence-based care in pain and symptom control.

For patients and their families, quality of life will be maximized in situations where the goals of symptom management and palliative care are valued. A good understanding of psychosocial stressors involved in cancer and palliative care will assist in good communication both with colleagues and with the patient and his or her family. This will result in expert symptom management and enhanced quality of life for all.

References

Barraclough J (1997) Depression, anxiety and confusion. British Medical Journal 315: 1365-1368.

Bottomley A (1997a) Cancer support groups – Are they effective? European Journal of Cancer 6: 11-17 .

Bottomley A (1997b) Psychosocial problems in cancer care: a brief review of common problems. Journal of Psychiatric and Mental Health Nursing 4: 323-331.

Bottorff JL, Gogag M, Engelberg-Lotzkar M (1995) Comforting: exploring the work of cancer nurses. Journal of Advanced Nursing 22: 1077-1084.

Brophy L, Sharp E (1991) Physical symptoms of biotherapy: a quality of life issue. Oncology Nursing Forum 18(suppl): 25-30.

Cervero F (1991) Visceral pain. In: Dubvier R, Gebhart FG, Bond MR (eds), Proceedings of the 5th World Conference on Pain. Amsterdam: Elsevier Science Publishers, pp. 216-226.

Cimprich B (1992) Attentional fatigue following breast cancer surgery. Research in Nursing and Health 15: 199-207.

Cimprich B (1993) Development of an intervention to restore attention in cancer patients. Cancer Nursing 16 : 83-92.

Clarke E, French B, Bilodeau M, Capasso V, Edwards A, Empolili J (1996) Pain management knowledge, attitudes and clinical practice: the impact of nurses' characteristics and education. Journal of Pain Symptom Management 11: 18-31.

Cook N (1999) Self-concept and cancer: understanding the nursing role. British Journal of Nursing 8: 318-324.

Cooley D (2000) Communication skills in palliative care. Professional Nurse 15: 602-605.

Copp G (1994) Palliative care nursing education: a review of research findings. Journal of Advanced Nursing 19: 552-557.

Corner J (1993) The impact of nurses encounters with cancer on their attitudes towards the disease. Journal of Clinical Nursing 2: 363-372.

Courtens AM, Stevens FCJ, Crebolder HFJM, Philipson H (1996) Longitudinal study on quality of life and social support in cancer patients. Cancer Nursing 19: 162-169.

Davitz LL, Davitz JR (1985) Culture and nurses' inference of suffering. In: Copp LA (ed.), Recent Advances in Nursing: Perspectives on pain. Edinburgh: Churchill Livingstone, pp. 17-28..

de Rond ME, de Wit R, Dam Van FS et al. (1999) Daily pain assessment: value for nurses and patients. Journal of Advanced Nursing 29: 436-444.

de Wit R, Van Dam F, Vielvoye-Kerkmeer A, Mattern C, Abu-Saad HH (1999) The treatment of chronic pain in a cancer hospital in the Netherlands. Journal of Pain and Symptom Management 17: 333-350.

Department of Health (1995) A policy framework for commissioning cancer care services. A report by the expert advisory group on cancer to the chief medical officers of England and Wales. London: DoH.

Dorepaal KL, Aaronson NK ,Van Dam FSAM (1989) Pain experience and pain management among hospitalised cancer patients. A clinical study. Cancer 63: 593-598.

Drayer RA, Henderson BS, Reidenberg M (1999) Barriers to better pain control in hospitalised patients. Journal of Pain and Symptom Management 17: 434-440.

Ernst E, Fialka V (1994) Ice freezes pain? A review of the clinical effectiveness of analgesic cold therapy. Journal of Pain and Symptom Management 9: 56-59 .

Faggerhaugh SY, Strauss A (1977) Politics of Pain Management. Staff-Patient Interaction. New York: Addison-Wesley.

Ferrell BA, Zichi Cohen M, Rhiner M, Rozek A (1991a) Pain as a metaphor for illness. Part II Family care givers management of pain. Oncology Nursing Forum 18: 1315-1321.

Ferrell BR, Ferrell BA, Rhiner M, Grant M (1991b) Cancer pain management. Postgraduate Medicine 67: 564-569.

Ferrell B, Dow K, Leigh S, Ly J, Gulasekarem P (1995) Quality of life in long term cancer survivors. Oncology Nursing Forum 22: 915-922.

Ferrell BR, Grant M, Dean GE, Funk B, Ly J (1996) 'Bone tired': the experience of fatigue and its impact on quality of life. Oncology Nursing Forum 23: 1539-1547.

Ferrell B, Dow K, Haberman M, Eaton L (1999) The meaning of life in cancer survivorship. Oncology Nursing Forum 26: 519-528.

Fieler V (1997) Side effects and quality of life issues in patients receiving high dose rate brachytherapy. Oncology Nursing Forum 24: 545-553.

Fordham M, Dunn S (1994) Alongside the Person in Pain. London: Baillière Tindall.

Fothergill-Bourbonnais F, Wilson Barnett J (1992) A comparative study of intensive therapy unit and hospice nurses' knowledge of pain management. Journal of Advanced Nursing 17: 362-372.

Franke AL, Theeuwen I (1994) Inhibition in expressing pain: a qualitative study among Dutch surgical breast cancer patients. Cancer Nursing 17: 193-199.

Franke AL, Garssen B, Abu Saad H, Grypdonck M (1996) Qualitative needs assessment prior to a continuing education program. Journal of Continuing Education for Nurses 27: 34-41.

Frankl V (1963) Man's Search for Meaning: An introduction to logotherapy. New York: Pocket Books.

Furstenburg C, Ahles TA, Whedon MB et al. (1998) Knowledge and attitudes of health care providers toward cancer pain management. A comparison of physicians, nurses and pharmacists in the state of New Hampshire. Journal of Pain and Symptom Management 15: 335-349.

Gordon M (1987) Nursing Diagnosis: Process and Application. New York: McGraw Hill.

Graffam S (1990) Pain content in the curriculum. A survey. Nurse Educator 15(1): 20-23.

Hanks GW (1994) Palliative medicine. Problem areas in pain and symptom management. Cancer Surveys 21: 1-3.

Hawthorn J, Redmond K (1998) Pain - Causes and Management. London: Blackwell Science.

Highfield MF (1992) Spiritual health of oncology patients nurse and patients perspectives. Cancer Nursing 15: 1-8 .

Hovi SL, Lauri S (1999) Patients' and nurses' assessment of cancer pain. European Journal of Cancer Care 8: 213-219.

Illich I (1976) Limits to Medicine: Medical nemesis. The expropriation of health. London: Marion Boyars.

Jacox A, Carr DB, Payne R et al. (1994) Management of Cancer Pain, Clinical Practice Guideline No 9, Agency for Health Care Policy and Research. AHCPR, Publication no 94-0592. Rockville, MD: AHCPR.

Jenkinson T (1996) The nurse as significant other for surgical patients. Professional Nurse 11: 651-652.

Klemm P, Miller M, Fernsler J (2000) Demands of illness in people treated for colorectal cancer. Oncology Nursing Forum 27: 635-639.

Kristjanson LJ, Avery L (1994) Vicarious pain: the family's perspective. Pain Management Newsletter 7(3): 1-2.

Larsen-Beck S (1991) The therapeutic use of music for cancer-related pain. Oncology Nursing Forum 18: 1327-1337.

McCaffery M (1990) Nursing approaches to non-pharmacological pain control. International Journal of Nursing Studies 27: 1-5.

McCaffery M, Beebe A (1989) Pain: A clinical manual for nursing practice. St Louis: CV Mosby Co.

McCaffery M, Ferrell B (1997) Nurses' knowledge of pain assessment and management: how much progress have we made? Journal of Pain and Symptom Management. 14: 175 -188.

McNamara P (1994) Massage for People with Cancer. London: Wandsworth Cancer Support Centre.

Magnusson K, Moller A, Ekman T, Wallgren A (1999) A qualitative study to explore the experiences of fatigue in cancer patients. European Journal of Cancer Care 8: 224-232.

Maleham K (1999) Promoting holistic well-being for people with cancer. MSc Dissertation, Leeds: Leeds Metropolitan University.

Menges LJ (1984) Pain: still an intriguing puzzle. Social Science and Medicine 19: 1257-1260.

Northouse PG, Northouse LL (1987) Communication and cancer: issues confronting patients, health professionals and family members. Journal of Psychosocial Oncology 5: 17-46.

Piper BF, Lidsey A, Dodd M (1987) Fatigue mechanisms in cancer patients: developing nursing theory. Oncology Nursing Forum 14(6): 17-23.

Porock D (1999) Fatigue. In: Aranda S, O'Conner M (eds), Palliative Care Nursing: A guide to practice. Melbourne: Ausmed Publications.

Redd WH, Montgomery GH, DuHamel KN (2001) Behavioral intervention for cancer treatment side effects. Journal of the National Cancer Institute. 93: 810-823.

Richardson A (1995) Fatigue in cancer patients: a review of the literature. European Journal of Cancer Care 4 : 20-32.

Richardson A, Ream E (1996) The experience of fatigue and other symptoms in patients receiving chemotherapy. European Journal of Cancer Care 5(suppl 2): 24-30.

Richardson A, Ream E (1999) From theory to practice: Designing interventions to reduce fatigue in patients with cancer. Oncology Nursing Forum 26: 1295-1303.

Rimer BK, Kedziera P, Levy MH (1992) The role of patient education in cancer pain. Hospice Journal 8: 171-191.

Ruckdeschel JC, Albrecht TL, Blanchard C, Hemmick RM (1996) Communication, accrual to clinical trials and the physician–patient relationship: implications for training programs. Journal of Cancer Education 11(2): 73-79.

Saunders C (1967) The Management of Terminal Illness. London: Hospice Medicine Publications.

Saunders P (1995) Depression in life threatening illness and its treatment. Nursing Times 91(11): 43–45.

Schon KC (1993) Awareness contexts and the construction of dying in the cancer treatment setting. Micro and macro levels in narrative analysis. In: Clark D (ed.), The Sociology of Death. Theory, Culture, Practice. Oxford: Blackwell.

Seers K (1987) Perceptions of pain. Nursing Times 83: 37–39.

Simpson M, Buckman R, Stewart M (1991) Doctor–patient communication: the Toronto consensus statement. British Medical Journal 303: 1385–1387.

Sindhu F (1996) Are non-pharmacological nursing interventions for the management of pain effective. A meta-analysis. Journal of Advanced Nursing 24: 1152–1159.

Thorne S (1985) The family cancer experience. Cancer Nursing 8: 285–291.

Thorne S (1999) Communication in cancer care: What science can and cannot teach us. Cancer Nursing 22: 370–378.

Twycross R (1994) Pain Relief in Advanced Cancer. Edinburgh: Churchill Livingstone.

Twycross R (1997) Symptom Management in Advanced Cancer, 2nd edn. Oxford: Radcliffe Medical Press.

Von Baeyer CL, Johnson MG, McMillan MJ (1984) Consequences of non-verbal expression of pain: patient distress and observer concern. Social Science and Medicine 19: 1319–1324.

Wainwright P (1985) Impact of hospital architecture on the patient in pain. In: Copp LA (ed.), Recent Advances in Nursing Perspectives on Pain. Edinburgh: Churchill Livingstone, pp. 46–61.

Wallace KG (1997) Analysis of recent literature concerning relaxation and imagery interventions for cancer pain. Cancer Nursing 20: 79–87.

Webb P (1992) Teaching patients and relatives. In: Tiffany R, Webb P (eds), Oncology for Nurses and Health Care Professionals, 2nd edn. Beaconsfield: Chapman & Hall, pp. 86–101.

Whitlock K (1999) Complementary therapies. In: Aranda S, O'Connor M (eds), Palliative Care Nursing. A guide to practice. Melbourne: Ausmed Publications, pp. 259–273.

Wilkinson S (1991) Factors which influence how nurses communicate with cancer patients. Journal of Advanced Nursing 16: 677–688.

Winningham M (1999) Fatigue. In: Yarbro C, Frogge M, Goodman M (eds), Cancer Symptom Management, 2nd edn. London: Jones & Bartlett, pp. 58–76.

Winningham M, Macvicar M, Johnson J (1985) Response of cancer patients on chemotherapy to a supervised exercise program. Medicine and Science in Sports and Exercise 17: 292.

Winningham ML, Nail LM, Burke MB et al. (1994) Fatigue and the cancer experience: the state of the knowledge. Oncology Nursing Forum 21: 23–36.

Woodruff R (1996) Cancer Pain. Melbourne: Asperula Pty Ltd.

World Health Organization (1994) Cancer Pain Relief. Geneva: WHO.

Zimmerman L, Pozehl B, Duncan K et al. (1989). Effects of music in patients who had chronic cancer pain. Western Journal of Nursing Research 11: 298–309.

Index